# The Inner Tradition of Yoga

# THE INNER TRADITION OF YOGA

A GUIDE TO YOGA PHILOSOPHY FOR THE CONTEMPORARY PRACTITIONER

Michael Stone

SHAMBHALA
BOSTON & LONDON
2008

Shambhala Publications, Inc.
Horticultural Hall
300 Massachusetts Avenue
Boston, Massachusetts 02115
www.shambhala.com



9 8 7 6 5 4 3 2 1
First Edition
Printed in the United States of America

♾ This edition is printed on acid-free paper that meets the American National Standards Institute Z39.48 Standard.
Distributed in the United States by Random House, Inc., and in Canada by Random House of Canada Ltd

Designed by Gopa & Ted2, Inc.

Library of Congress Cataloging-in-Publication Data
Stone, Michael.
The inner tradition of yoga: a guide to yoga philosophy for the contemporary practitioner / Michael Stone.
p. cm.
Includes bibliographical references and index.
ISBN 978-1-59030-569-0 (pbk.: alk. paper)
1. Yoga. I. Title.
B132.Y6S764 2008
181'.45—dc22
2007048880

"I do not know just what it is that I am like. I wander about concealed and wrapped in thought."

*—Rig-Veda*

# Contents

# Foreword

FOR YOGA, these are the best of times, yet in some ways, these are the worst of times. The explosion in information technology is bringing people and their cultures, ideas, languages, religions, and businesses together at an exciting and disconcerting pace. So far, no one culture, no one religion, no one government is able to define an absolute frame of reference to organize the whole thing.

Spreading almost like mushrooms with the eclectic world culture of multinationals, Internet cafes, and Starbucks is the practice of yoga. There is something naturally appealing about the yoga postures to all types of people. Approaching reality through the immediate physicality of the body, the senses, and the breath skips right around religious, cultural, and national prejudice, and brings out a love of the best and most beautiful in everything. This draws people to yoga so that there are enthusiastic, sincere, and educated yoga practitioners in even remote corners of Asia, the Middle East, Europe, and all of the Americas. Yoga has something remarkably universal about it. It is practically generic in its mysticism, which in its initial appeal to such a wide audience does not cast an oppressive net of a single belief, framework, or god-concept over the open and indeterminate process of living intelligence. There is still an innocence and naivety to the openness and enthusiasm shown worldwide for yoga. Can we keep the innocence as we become wise enough to see with love through the wily ways of our own egos? Or will that innocence be exploited by all of the profiteering, proselytizing, seducing, and reducing done by our egos to avoid true yoga? Can our yoga survive the remarkable rate of its own expansion? Will the potent and ancient tradition live through its commercial success? These remain open questions for yoga enthusiasts on both the personal and the collective levels.

It is completely understandable why there is such a strong tendency to take the active ingredient out of yoga, to package it to please and to sell, to avoid the very heart of yoga and, thereby, to avoid reality. Genuine yoga exposes the insubstantiality and emptiness of our self-image, which allows us to see the insubstantiality and emptiness of everything. Eventually remarkable courage, commitment, and compassion arise from yoga practice and, through those, a wonderful insight and joy. Yoga is far nicer than anything we could have wanted or bargained for. We simply have not been able to wrap our minds around it, and so before investigating it on its own terms, we are selling it unopened and untasted in the spiritual marketplace. The traditional context for yoga, awakening to the simple truth of impermanence, to universal death, is all that has been missing. This is what awakens our compassion and shows us the interconnectedness not only of all beings, but of techniques, styles, and viewpoints. It sobers the mind and wakes us up from spiritual pride and materialism.

Yoga has always been, and continues to be, subtle and impossible to express literally. Like love, it is taught with metaphor and poetry, with patterned practice and ecstatic release. Occasionally, and always in bad taste, the ego can trick us into imagining that our own specialized forms and languages have achieved universal status, when in fact they remain painfully provincial and riddled with blind spots. At any time, any yoga practitioner can grasp their practice form and language as literal and miss out on what is much more intelligent and pleasing. As humans with egos we can and frequently do mess up even the subtle and beautiful. Now our yoga is hitting the fan of the modern world. The variety of viewpoints, of techniques and styles, the attitudes and philosophies form a colorful array of trends mixed from the best and worst of modern cultures from all around the world. On one hand, there are new extreme styles of raunchy party yoga, cult narcissism, condescending asceticism. This adoration of the ego is forming a path of competition and vanity. On the other hand, with so much information and cross-cultural linking, there are breathtaking new ways and languages for teaching and ever more refined forms of an art of a yoga worthy of passing on to others.

Michael Stone has given us a true gift, which allows us to approach the practices and philosophies of yoga from the place where their variety makes sense. He lets us begin where we are, surrounded by the situations of our heart. Our relationships and our beliefs about the world have a direct effect on the deep sensations in our body that link into emotion and perception. The link between the mind and the body, between the *citta* and the *prāṇa,* forms the axiom around which many internal yoga practices revolve. Observing sensation closely through mindfulness of the breath reveals the vibratory and impermanent nature of things and allows the deconditioning of the mind from habitual patterns of response and association with those same sensations and feelings. *The Inner Tradition of Yoga* allows us to begin practicing on the deepest level before we commit to a viewpoint, a belief system, or a style. This psychological approach to yoga takes us straight into the heart of the misperceptions about who and what we are. To enter philosophy or yoga technique deeply, we must start grounded psychologically. We can then bypass the ego games that we might play when the subject of yoga is presented as difficult philosophy or as a physically stimulating and challenging art.

*The Inner Tradition of Yoga* looks at yoga as it is and then shows us a simple, compassionate way through the variety, complexity, and challenges that face us in our personal practice and, collectively, as we create a culture based in the most universal principles of yoga. It approaches yoga practice and philosophy from the immediate experience of our

# A Note on Pronunciation of Sanskrit Terms

THE TRANSLITERATION of Sanskrit into English is always an approximation at best. The short *a* in Sanskrit is pronounced like the *u* in the English word *but,* and the long *ā* is pronounced like the *a* in father.

In terms of the family of consonants, an easy approximation is possible by pronouncing *c* as in *church, j* as in jump, *ṣ* as in *shut, s* as in *sun,* and *ś* as something halfway between the previous two. Aspirated consonants are quite distinct: *bh* as in *cab horse, dh* as in *madhouse, gh* as in *doghouse, ph* as in *top hat,* and *th* as in *goatherd.* The letter *ṛ* is a vowel, pronounced somewhere between *ri* as in *rim* and *er* as in *mother.*

The transliterated letter and character *ñ,* found in a word like *Patañjali,* can be pronounced like the *ni* in *onion,* and when found with the letter *j* in the word *prajña* can be pronounced like the *gn* in the word *igneous.*

Sometimes I pluralize a word like *yama* by simply adding an *s,* resulting in *yama*s, which is unacceptable for the academic or Sanskritist, but essential for simple reading for those unfamiliar with the language. Unless otherwise attributed, the translations are my own. Try your best pronouncing these new sounds—as you get used to them, they open the palette and help concentrate the mind. Enjoy!

# The Inner Tradition of Yoga

# Introduction

IN A SMALL second-floor room at the Marpa House in Boulder, Colorado, several hours after we finished an intense practice of back bending, the eighty-three-year-old Indian yoga master Sri K. Pattabhi Jois held court for three hours, inviting students to sit down and ask him questions. I sat at the side of the room, eager to participate in discussion and also interested in observing how he fielded questions from students in an entirely different cultural context than Mysore, India. In his typically quiet way, smiling and wondering if he knew any students from previous meetings, Guruji sat in front of a Tibetan *thangka* painting that draped behind him like a saffron moon.

I was struck by the variety of cultures in the room that day. Eager American Hatha Yoga practitioners, sitting in a room with a Brahmin, who himself was sitting in front of a colorful Tibetan Buddhist painting depicting the Buddhist deity of compassion. Outside the door, Guruji's host and respected American yoga teacher Richard Freeman greeted visitors, who would take off their shoes, bow down to Guruji's feet, and look up at him waiting for one of his familiar sayings, for instance "One by one, all is coming." Barefoot and eager to meet this foreign Indian yoga master, students sat cross-legged on velvet cushions and graciously bowed to him before sitting up with spines in perfect posture.

Guruji smiled, sometimes posing for a photograph and at other moments becoming a touch shy. Students filed through the room all afternoon, Guruji's attention unwavering.

I was surprised to hear most students primarily asking simple questions related to physical postures, to which he seemed indifferent. "How long will it take to practice a good back bend?" one student asked; Guruji smiled without reply. Another student asked if Guruji could recommend a way to practice forward bends with less pressure on his knees. Guruji replied with a much-awaited and by now famous line, "Many lifetimes, all is coming."

Yet when people would ask him questions about movements of energy, how to work with the mind, *kuṇḍalinī*, or esoteric texts, he would light up and begin quoting *śāstras*, traditional texts, memorized with depth and accuracy. Unless one knew Sanskrit, his responses were vague and incomprehensible. When Guruji was excited about a question, he almost never answered in English.

I was struck by the variety of sources from which he quoted: the *Yoga-Sutra, Bhagavad Gītā, Chāndogya Upaniṣad, Ṛg-Veda, Yoga Taravali, Hatha Yoga Pradīpika,* and a few other Sanskrit references with which I was unfamiliar.

As the afternoon rolled on and the meeting became more intimate, I noticed that Pattabhi Jois touched his heart every time he spoke of breathing, self, or god. At one point, I raised my hand and asked him this: "Guruji, every time you talk about breathing, God, or the present moment, you touch your heart. Can you say something about that?"

He paused a moment as he scanned the room, raised his glance in my direction, and enthusiastically responded.

"When students breathing," he said, "trying to practice yoga, breathing into heart. Students breathe into heart looking for God right here. God is in heart. Students want to find God but not finding God. Students breathe into heart finding enemies."

"'Enemies?'" I asked. "What do you mean 'enemies'? Enemies in the heart?"

"Students finding enemies in heart. Six enemies," he said. "*Kāma, krodha, moha, lobha, mada, mātsarya.*"

"What do these words mean?" I asked. He could not find the English equivalent. Someone mentioned that maybe he meant jealousy, envy, and possibly greed. Another thought he spoke of hatred.

Then someone else asked a question, and the room was onto another topic.

Over the next few days, I couldn't stop thinking about these six enemies. What were they? What prevents the heart from opening? Of what are these six enemies symptomatic? What is the relationship between breathing and the divine? How did these enemies act as obstacles to freedom? I had many questions but did not have another chance to ask Pattabhi Jois, since his two-week teaching session was coming to an end. All that I was able to understand at the time was that the six enemies referred to the six poisons: kāma ("desire"), krodha ("anger"), moha ("delusion"), lobha ("greed"), mada ("envy"), mātsarya ("sloth"). These six poisons are symptomatic of a heart unsatisfied, a life characterized by suffering.

We begin practicing yoga postures in an effort to relieve suffering and find a way to meet life with less effort and more flexibility. Yoga is a path out of suffering. But what we find after our initial foray or honeymoon period is a matrix of psychological and physical holding patterns that have captured our minds and bodies within tightly conditioned parameters.

Some time later, I had the opportunity to ask Pattabhi Jois how to work with the poisons of desire, anger, delusion, greed, envy, and sloth, to which he responded, in an answer that would radically change my understanding of yoga and psychology in general, "Understanding the heart by understanding the five *kleṣa*s. Knowing five kleṣas, no more poison; no more poison, no more *duḥkha*."

What Pattabhi Jois describes with his antidote of the five kleṣas is a reference to the *Yoga-Sutra* attributed to the sage Patañjali, which describes in detail the five factors that keep us spinning in the conditioned wheel of suffering. The symptoms of unmediated desire, laziness, greed, envy, and other poisons are manifestations of deeper psychological factors, namely the five kleṣas. These five factors that contribute to our discontent concisely sum up the essential teachings of yoga psychology. Getting down to the roots of suffering and its corresponding symptoms requires an investigation of the five kleṣas. All practices of yoga, including meditation, breathing techniques, ethics, postures, and devotional practices, bring the practitioner into contact with the core of the heart. Along this path of the heart one is sure to find obstacles. One cannot work with the body without also working with the mind, because when we work with the symptoms of discontent, we begin to see that physiology and psychology are inseparable. The five kleṣas describe yoga psychology in a nutshell.

*Avidyā* can be defined as "not being with life as it is." It comes from the root *vidyā,* which in Latin becomes *vidéo,* refined into English as *video,* meaning "to see." When you put the prefix *a* before a word in Sanskrit, it turns that word into its opposite; in this case *a* denotes *not* seeing things clearly. Avidyā is descriptive of a state of mind and body unengaged with the present moment, unaware of reality as it really is.

*Raga* (attachment) is the desire to repeat pleasurable experience. *Dveṣa* (aversion) is the leaning away from what is unpleasurable. Moment after moment, day after day, we flip-flop back and forth between raga and dveṣa, reactive patterns in mind and body that keep us from being present by trying to either cling to pleasure or avert displeasure.

*Asmitā* is the construction of the stories of "I, me, and mine." Asmitā refers to the construction of a self around which our perceptual world pivots. Whenever there is either attachment or aversion, there is the birth of a story of "me." The stories of "I, me, and mine" are generated when we identify consciousness with pure awareness and thus create a gap in our experience between what is actually occurring and the deep-seated need to filter what is happening through stories about ourselves.

Constantly perceiving our experience through the lens of "me" creates separation from the nature of what is arising in the present moment and consequently gives rise to *duḥkha,* a feeling of lack and alienation.

*Abhiniveśa* is the fear of letting go of the story of "I, me, mine." The fear of death entails more than the loss of this body, rather it goes to the heart of our deepest attachment: the stories of "me" and the corresponding belief in a substantial and enduring self. Abhiniveśa is the thirst for further existence. It is the fear of letting go of all forms of attachment and aversion. Why? Because the construction of self creates separation from that which is occurring in the present by splitting experience into "me" and "that," subject and object. When we let go of the continual construction of a self or even the need to be a "somebody," then we are free to be who we are. When we are completely ourselves, we forget about needing to be the center of our perceptual world and thus we can take in others and our environment with greater sensitivity, compassion, and openness.

In essence, Pattabhi Jois described what many yoga practitioners experience as practice matures, namely, that one cannot work exclusively on the physical aspects of yoga without also working with the psychological dimension of practice. To leave out the role of psychology in shaping and determining our way of being in the world is to bypass the deeper layers of yoga practice—layers that ultimately cause us to repeat habitual rounds of discontent and distress. We can experience, without doubt, certain physical transformations that occur when we practice yoga postures, but to drop into deeper holding patterns requires an attention span without preference or aversion—a mind that can be present with whatever shows up in the field of awareness. Otherwise, our deeper holding patterns produce recurring symptoms, described in Sanskrit as *granthi,* which literally refers to the knots of mind and body. These knots are known initially through the symptoms of discontent, namely the six poisons.

The poisons, when left unconscious, lead to unskillful actions, which generate *karma*, the infallible activity of cause and effect that reverberates through each individual and the web of life as a whole. Actions stemming from the symptomatic conditions described by Pattabhi Jois as "enemies in the heart" give rise to suffering both internally and externally. Pattabhi Jois was saying, in very few words, that all forms of suffering—physical and psychological—are caused by these five kleṣas and that when one investigates the way in which these kleṣas operate, both on and off the yoga mat, the path of the heart opens up. If the kleṣas are not studied and deconstructed, one by one, the symptoms of dissatisfaction dominate our modes of perception and our basic actions. All symptoms assert themselves because they need attention. Rather than approaching the six poisons as symptoms that we need to be rid of with a problem-solving attitude, we instead look deeply into the underlying causes of these symptoms, namely the five kleṣas, and in doing so, we turn the symptoms of our suffering into the very path itself.

When Pattabhi Jois touched his heart in a simple gesture of breathing and then went on to describe the enemies that reside in the heart, which are nothing other than the symptoms that manifest when we don't see things as they are, I realized that yoga practice matures, not by adding more and more spectacular postures but by simply paying attention to the movements of the breath in the space of the heart and the role of the mind with the body, not apart from it. The five kleṣas describe the essence of yoga: a path of freedom from our habitual cycles of discontent.

# 1. *Vidyā*

## SEEING THINGS AS THEY ARE

YOGA BEGINS in the present moment, and the present moment begins in silence. From that silence, words are born. In the *Yoga-Sutra* attributed to Patañjali (third century B.C.E.), considered to be one of the core texts of yoga psychology, we begin with a simple sentence: "*Atha yoganusāsanam.*" This is translated as "in the present moment is the teaching of yoga."

The *Yoga-Sutra* is not a speculative text on philosophy or metaphysics, nor does it offer us a theology of creation or a final comment on what's in store for us after death. Creation and death coexist in sequence with the arising and passing away of each moment. Every inhalation is a birth and the end of every exhalation is a small death. In each consecutive moment, over and over again, the universe arises and passes away on the thread of a breath cycle.

The first word in the *Yoga-Sutra—atha*—literally means "now," "what is here in this moment." Yoga begins in the present moment. Yoga *is* the present moment. We could more concisely translate this opening line as: "Yoga begins now." The teachings of yoga orient us toward this very moment, rendering the future invisible and the past no longer in reach. Many scholars and practitioners translate *yoga* as a manifestation of the verb *yuj*—"to unite"—which turns yoga into something one does, a form of willful activity. In thinking that yoga is the act of uniting one thing with another (breath with movement, body with mind, self with other), we confuse yoga with the doing of yoga. When we use the term in this way (as in "I'm going to practice yoga"), we confuse the techniques or the technology of practice with the experience of yoga. In every unfolding moment, in any meeting with any person, even in meeting ourselves, everything is complete. This completeness doesn't mean that everything is put together in some master plan. It means that everything is interdependent and that yoga is not something we seek outside of ourselves or a willful attempt at union, but the recognition, in the present moment, of the unification of life. The inherent interconnectedness of existence reveals what in philosophical terms we call "nondualism"—the collapse of separation between subject and object. When we experience relaxed openness and attentive awareness, the world reveals its inherent completeness. When we move through the world, "concealed and wrapped in thought," there is no direct contact with reality and we know not "who or what" we are. Yoga begins with the gesture of a gentle bow in service of the present moment.

Yoga is a way of being and a mode of existing. Existence is a play of interconnectedness, and the more we clarify our perception and ways of organizing our experiences, the more openness and compassion we bring to the profound and sometimes confusing undertaking of being in the world. The authentic practice of yoga is an unremitting attention to present experience, whether in mind, body, or heart, with a baby on the hip, making breakfast, or balancing the breath in a headstand.

According to yoga philosophy and psychology, the only place to begin an investigation of yoga—or of anything for that matter—is the present moment, because *this* is all that is actually occurring. The future has not yet arisen and the past is passed; the only thing there is to investigate and the only way to begin paying attention is within this very experience as it unfolds right now, right here. That is why an investigation into the nature of reality and the true nature of the mind begins in this life, this body, and this moment; it can't begin with an investigation of anything other than the here and now of our moment-to-moment, verifiable experience. The mind, with all its fantastic, distracted, and creative potential, is so used to weaving conceptions and preferences all over the present moment that we are often relating not to what is actually occurring in life but reacting to life with our likes and dislikes. That is why psychological inquiry in the service of awakening begins with what is happening in the here and now—a form of present-centered attention with acceptance.

The mind has a hard time watching anything for very long, especially its own workings. The mind has a hard time being present as the breath moves in the body or as sensations arise and fall away in different yoga poses, and as a result, we are not often here most of the time. This is true not just in relationship with our own bodies and emotions but interpersonally as well. Other people interrupt our ideas about the way things are supposed to be. This interruption is precisely what yoga is all about: becoming flexible enough to have our preconceptions and our elaborative tendencies interrupted. We usually discover a lot more in the silent space between thoughts than through all the interpretations, ideas, and views our minds generate. Moments of psychological stillness remind us that there are ways of knowing other than intellectual or habitual. Yoga practice, both on and off the mat, opens up the heart by revealing our patterns of grasping and inflexibility. This practice leaves no stone unturned. Through a disciplined and appropriately designed yoga practice, we not only see clearly our conditioned ways of living but we learn how to let go of those patterns so that our questions radically outnumber our answers. When we are open, and our habitual psychological and physical ways of being are suspended, we arrive in the present moments of life free to respond with an open and creative heart.

Yoga is an investigation into who we are and what we are. We are not just investigating our everyday neuroses (though sometimes part of the path), nor are we philosophically investigating metaphysics (again, only a minor mode of inquiry)—we are looking into the nature of existence by starting with mind, breath, and body. This requires the ability to be patient and accepting of what is occurring in our mind-body so we can see something clearly enough to study it. But how do we study our own mind? How do we investigate our own body? How can an eye see itself or the tip of a fingernail touch itself or the ear hear itself? Our perception is always hiding a shadow. We can never, it seems, see something in its entirety, there is always a blind spot in our perceptual field.

We perceive our experience—and the entire universe—by labeling "things" that seem to be "out there" and "solid." And what becomes solid "out there" allows "me" to feel solid as well. I have a body in space and time. When I feel my body internally, I feel the breath, muscles, and bones, even the fascia. But I can't locate my body exactly. When I say "bone," there is not only a feeling but an image as well. The image comes from a skeleton I once saw in a lab. Then I feel the breath but can't tell exactly where it begins or ends, or where it starts at the nostrils, or its precise place of exit. When I eat a carrot, I cannot tell, once chewed, where the carrot ends and where "I" begin.

The body, on further subjective meditation, is not a static thing; it's primarily a concept layered over other concepts with some changing sensations, feelings, perceptions, and breath mixed up among them. I can feel a form that I'd call "body," but I can't say where it is or what it is. I don't know for certain where it begins or ends, especially with my eyes closed. The body is not an actual thing that one can study—the body and the one who studies it are one. The observer and the body cannot be separated. Whether we examine the inner world of mind and body or the outer world of "things," we cannot find in our perception any "thing" that actually exists. If I say, "Show me your ego," could you do that? Where is your ego? You know you have an ego, but how do you know this? Mostly we know through inference—I can tell when I am self-centered—but that is a few steps back from direct experience. I cannot find the mechanism called "ego," nor can I remove it. The ground is groundless. How do we determine what we are and what we are not? If we are to map a perimeter of our existence, where do we draw the line between where we end and where what is external to us begins? The fact is that the common distinctions we make between things is the very mechanism that creates "things" in the first place. Duality, the creating of a self "in here" that perceives an object "out there," always creates separateness and alienation. Dualism is self-constructed; it's not built into reality as it presents itself. This takes us straight to the heart of yoga practice: yoga is the inherent union and interconnectedness of all existence before we split things up into subject, object, or any method of categorization.

If dualistic perception is so deeply embedded in our psychological makeup, where does one begin? For the yoga practitioner, one begins right here in this moment. Whether through the practices of *prāṇāyāma,* mantra, *āsana,* or ethics, the systems of yoga arise out of and point to the same thing: the present moment. Even in the visualization of a breathing pattern or a meditation on sound, one dissolves the outer environment into the object of concentration. Then the object of concentration collapses into an experience of being completely centered and still. This stillness is a point of nothingness, yet is also everything. It is being with nobody there. It is being so fully present in an action (or nonaction) that you don't need to create a self. When we live authentically, we are not simultaneously creating a sense of "I, me, or mine"; we are simply being our selfless self.

In yoga posture practice we dissolve the technique of moving the body into pure feeling and then dissolve the mind into that deep experience of feeling. Then, that is all that is there. In chanting, as another example, we dissolve seed syllables into pure sound, and then sound into quiet, and then quiet into stillness, and then stillness becomes nothing other than a contented mind that is open and receptive, sharp and still. When the mind returns to this natural state, anything can arise in mind, body, and heart, and there is no pushing or pulling, just arising and dissolving, one form becoming, in turn, another. Again, in these various techniques, the essence of the practice is what the technique is pointing toward rather than the technique itself. But since the mind has a hard time becoming centered enough to relax into a state of stillness, we need technique to help us along. The point of practice is not the goal but the way that the different stages of the path propel is into a more open and sincere way of being. This sincerity of being (*karuṇā*) is the ongoing result of a healthy yoga practice. If our practice is creating flexibility of the body without a corresponding flexibility of the heart, we need to redress the way we conceive of and engage in practice.

This book is about how to cultivate a yoga practice, what constitutes a yoga practice, how to recognize and work with the different stages on the path, and how to keep the tradition of yoga a living tradition through committed practice and critical engagement. On a heart level, this book is about the cultivation of patience, honesty, nonviolence, wisdom, and the ability to meet life as it occurs from moment to moment without habitual forms of clinging. Whether you are just beginning your practice or you have studied deeply in a particular system, you should be able to find here some suggestions and encouragement for deepening your practice.

There are two themes in this book: (1) The essence of yoga teaches us that all forms of clinging create suffering. Nothing can be owned as "I, me, and mine." And (2) a disciplined and appropriate practice leaves no stone unturned. A broad understanding of yoga theory integrated with specific practices takes the formal techniques of yoga to deeper levels but also brings yoga off the mat, out of the meditation hall and into the tangled world of our interpersonal relationships, our habitual psychological holding patterns, and the complexity of ethical action. This book moves back and forth between these two themes—practice and letting go—by weaving together theory and responsive action.

Along with the primary theme of letting go of our attachments, especially to self-image, this book attempts to bridge the gap in contemporary yoga between practice and theory. My aim is to not only reconcile theory and practice but to explore how both theory and practice come alive when integrated in daily life. So, unlike much of the usual teaching methodology, this book focuses on words rather than postures, suggestions rather than instructions, interpretations based on tradition rather than appropriation or idealization. Within the words on these pages, see if you can listen with your heart rather than your intellect. We are used to hearing what we usually call "theory" with the intellectual mind. When ideas in yoga are listened to with just the intellect, they remain at a distance from the heart, and in this way we can miss the essence and wisdom of this practice and how it has the ability to challenge and open up the heart. Yoga is about how we can take in teachings and put them into practice; how we can sit openly with mind and body, breath, and stillness, and then let them spread out in the wide-open world of nature and other human beings. Yoga opens us up to a state of being where the world passes transparently through us.

Like the inhalation that arises and the exhalation that passes away, every moment is in itself a moment of creation followed by dissolution. Like the rising and falling of the breath, or the dawning and setting of the sun, this book follows that same rhythm. The first chapters begin with a description and definition of yoga and from there describe the various paths of practice. Like the top end of an inhale or the high-noon sun, the first part of this book moves toward a description of the psychology and energetic aspects of yoga. Descending from there, we explore the teachings of impermanence, emptiness, and death, which in essence bring us into direct engagement with life. This cycle naturally completes itself, because contemplating impermanence and death connects us with the present moment, which is where yoga begins.

Yoga begins with an honest meeting of our present experience, which means seeing as best we can all aspects of ourselves and our world, including what is most difficult or painful. The outer reflection of our created life does not always provide an accurate reading of the state of the inner life. How much suffering have we felt through our inability to tolerate and live in the midst of change? How much difficulty do we experience from our reactions to the interactivity of feelings, thoughts, movements in the body, and memory? The sense of ourselves at an innermost level is entangled with our reactions to the gross and subtle movements in the mind and body. The mind and body belong to a moment-to-moment process, not to our clinging habits nor to the ways we want things to be or wish they were. Yoga is freedom from this satisfaction-dissatisfaction cycle we call "me" and "mine." And the path through this ongoing cycle of habit begins in the present moment, which originates in our perceptual field of mind and body.

In the *Yoga-Sutra,* a textbook on yoga as a psychological practice, Patañjali initiates the path of yoga with two first steps: practice (*abhyāsa*) and letting go (*vairāgya*). Cultivating more wholesome intentions and actions of body, speech, and mind, and letting go of historical and ensnaring attitudes, is a constant throughout the entire path. Cultivating positive qualities and letting go of negative factors in our psychophysical makeup gives us a clear starting point for our practice, without which we risk getting lost in the futility of undirected movement. It is easy to engage in a language of freedom and impermanence or think that just completing a regimented sequence of yoga postures is going to free up our deepest holding patterns. It is something else to feel impermanence, freedom, and deep kindness in our bones. We can only know a grounded, flexible, and free life when we commit to practice and cultivate the skill of letting go.

After several years of consistent practice, a gap emerged between the theory I was studying and the protocol of posture technique, breathing, and meditation I was practicing, so I began asking questions. The first questions were broad questions about how texts related to one another and why certain practices, such as the contemporary yoga sequences commonly found in yoga studios, were not represented in ancient texts. Then the questions become more personal, and related to the absence of psychological understanding in yoga communities and the eventual vanity that comes on the heels of superficial practice. As I began questioning what I was practicing, slowly I felt that everything I knew and all of the practices I had been working on began to slip away. The questions led first to doubt and then to a state of not knowing why I was practicing or what practice actually was. I saw around me people accomplishing great feats of flexibility and wonderful posture practices, but those same practices did not guarantee a commensurate opening of the heart. Perfection in yoga poses did not guarantee psychological or spiritual insight.

What do we aspire to in practice? What motivates our practice? What is the reason for practice? Some say we practice for no reason, but human experience seems always constructed within the context of purpose or meaning. How does one live a good life? What is enlightenment? Is yoga just about physical accomplishment, and if not, why are the ethical and psychological underpinnings of yoga so underspoken? Does one have to finally hold their own heels in back bends, practice arm balances in full lotus, or is there some other test for the liberative validity of practice?

# 2. Embracing Suffering

IN THE MEDIEVAL TEXT on yoga known as the *Yoga Vāsiṣṭa,* Rama is asked by his father why he has a heavy heart and why he is having such a hard time in his mind and with his body. With low eyes and a sunken chest, Rama responds by saying,

> My heart has begun to question: what do people call happiness and can it be had in the ever-changing objects of this world? All beings in this world take birth only to die and die to be born. I do not perceive any meaning at all in these transient phenomena . . . . Unrelated beings come together; the mind conjures up a relationship between them. Everything in this world is dependent on the mind and one's attitude. On examination, the mind is unreal, it cannot be found. But we are bewitched by it. This is suffering.[1]

The king, who is also present for the conversation between Rama and his father, responds first by saying that Rama's perception of his condition is the root of the problem.

> Rama's condition is not the result of delusion, the king continues, but is full of wisdom and points to enlightenment.[2]

When the sages, ministers, and community of the court hear this exchange, they stop their doings and become completely still. They hear in Rama's flaming words their own doubts, fears, and misunderstandings. The royal family, citizens, pets, caged birds, horses in the royal stables, and even the heavenly musicians are silenced by the way Rama gives expression to their deepest fears, hopes, and desires. How does one work with the inherent suffering of being human?

Yoga not only begins in the present moment (*atha*) but begins also with the recognition of suffering, stress, discontent, and dissatisfaction that characterizes much of our moment-to-moment experience. The characteristics of suffering appear in the heart as poisons. Here is how Pattabhi Jois describes it:

> In the yoga śāstra it is said that god dwells in our heart in the form of light, but this light is covered by six poisons: kāma, krodha, moha, lobha, mātsarya, and mada. These are desire, anger, delusion, greed, envy and sloth."[3]

Not only does Rama articulate a universal truth about human suffering, but the king responds in a surprising way. Rather than asking Rama to further explain his anguish and discontent, he describes Rama's problem as an error of perception. It is not that Rama is caught in delusion, but rather that Rama is deluded about his own delusion. His suffering is not the problem, it's that he doesn't see that his suffering is the source of wisdom and the actual path to enlightenment. Rather than treating his anguish as something to be expelled, the king infers, anguish is a recognition that the path has opened. The king does not define enlightenment in this first chapter, nor does he offer a series of techniques to follow to find freedom from torment. Instead he offers Rama a complete reversal, a counterperception that defines the path of yoga as embracing one's suffering and, in so doing, uses complete acceptance as a starting point for practice.

In the same way that Pattabhi Jois describes the enemies of the heart as the factors that create suffering, he also points to the heart with his own breath as a means of saying that the path begins in the heart, the body, the mind, even with their enemies. In the language of devotional *Bhakti* yoga, it is said that the cure of the symptom begins with love. This is not personal love in the sense of a new-age sensitivity or empathic technique but rather the impersonal force of love that heals by extending itself to the most interrupted, broken, and ruined parts of ourselves.

Like Rama, or many other well-known characters that populate Indian literature (I think also of Arjuna in the *Bhagavad Gītā*), I came to yoga practice because I was suffering. Most practitioners come to yoga to deal with the myriad forms of upset, stress, and lack. For many, that stress may be recognizable in the daily grind of work, difficulties in relationships, or dissatisfaction in the form of tight hamstrings. But some level of dissatisfaction brings us to yoga, however that is defined and described, if at all, consciously or unconsciously, and its expression and manifestation are unique for everyone. One of the key teachings of yoga, as described in the *Sāṇkhya Karika* of Ishvarakṛṣṇa, is that life is characterized by duḥkha, suffering. This is one of the central tenets of Kṛṣṇa's teaching to Arjuna in the *Bhagavad Gītā,* the king's comments to Rama in the *Yoga Vāsiṣṭa,* Patañjali's starting point in the *Yoga-Sutra,* and the Buddha's first noble truth: life is characterized by dissatisfaction and pervasive lack.

"There is just enough suffering to get you in the door," I often tell yoga students, in order to remind them of why they are in class, "so that is our starting point." Difficulty begets faith. Faith in yoga implies a sense of yearning. What are we yearning for, what do we seek to be free of? For many of us, the longing to practice yoga has to do with aspiring to a life free of habitual patterns of conditioning. If we seek any kind of transcendence, we are always looking for something we do not yet know. So faith is a movement beyond what we currently feel is constricting, and in that sense it is a yearning. At some level, we all yearn to overcome places in which there is constriction, lack, and discontent. Faith in practice requires not a theological commitment but rather an interest in one's discontent and how to bring it to an end.

Longing is not to be dismissed as a form of attachment but an inevitable part of what keeps us going. Of course, it can get mixed up with the projects of the ego, but there is an inherent longing to see through the limitations of the ego. We long to know the nature of things and to connect and be grounded in relationship with something larger than our ideas of ourselves. We know so much about so many things, but what do we really know when pressed with anguish or pain? What do we learn about our character when up against the truth of change, the truth of death, the truth of suffering?

When I began practicing yoga, the first classes I attended, in the basement of a library, consisted of little more than sitting still and watching the cycles of the breath. I had a hard time sitting still for more than one breath cycle, and by the time I reached the top of an inhalation, my mind was on to something else. The teacher instructed us to notice the breath and whatever physical and mental states were coming and going. Eventually, I began to notice the ways the mind and body were deeply conditioned with patterns of reactivity. Before she had us move our bodies, the teacher required that we could sit still and notice the feeling of simple breathing and the mind's tendency to escape those simple sensations.

"All of human unhappiness is due to the inability to sit still in a room alone," writes philosopher Blaise Pascal in his treatise on the human condition.[4] Too often, our first response to sense data is to think about it, and when caught in our thinking, we begin to withdraw into a representational reality constructed in our own mind. The miracle of yoga is what Patañjali calls *viveka,* the ability to distinguish the difference between self-centered thinking, along with the separation it creates, and the ongoing nondual experience of being in touch with life.

Inextricably linked to the teaching of duḥkha is the way that suffering continues in cycles, like a wheel spinning out of balance. This turning of the wheel of duḥkha is called *saṁsāra.* Saṁsāra is a metaphor for meaninglessness. It refers to the endless cycle of birth, death, and rebirth. But the concept of the cycle of birth and rebirth is not simply a carryover from Indian cultural attitudes about the possibility of future or past lives, but rather the birth, death, and rebirth of our sense of self from moment to moment. Each moment of experience, whether in stillness or in reactivity, sets up the pattern for the next consecutive moment, and our ability to skillfully meet each and every moment with open and undivided attention is possible to astonishing degrees. This moment conditions the next.

Psychological rebirth is a metaphor for being born into a conditioned existence. Yoga practice is about breaking free of the cyclic force of habitual activity and distorted mental and emotional forces that drive us to act in ways that maintain suffering. While this is not an image of hell, per se, it is thought that saṁsāra and duḥkha are one and the same. Suffering is a product of conditioned existence.

Sometimes turning to the imaginative and mythical tales of India helps us better understand the workings of the mind. Carl Jung reminds us that "mythology is where the psyche 'was' before psychology made it an object of investigation."[5] In another tale from the *Yoga Vāsiṣṭa,* Sikhidhavaja asks Kumbha what the nature of the mind is so that he can finally put it to rest. "Tell me the exact nature of the mind," Sikhidhavaja asks, "then I can know how to abandon its habits so that they do not arise again and again."

Kumbha responds by saying that all conditioned patterns (saṁsāra) exist in the mind and body as *vāsanā*s (memories, subtle impressions of the past, conditioning). "In fact," he says, "the subtle impressions from the past and the mind itself are synonymous." Most mind states are made of habits, and those very habits add up to what we call "a life," though such an existence is superficial and alienating. Yoga technology is a means of becoming free of our mind's habitual grasping and contractions.

"How does one let go of the repetition of past experience?" asks Sikhidhavaja, wondering if there is a way beyond self-reference and its resulting discontent. "The end of relating to each experience through the filter of saṁsāra," Kumbha says, "occurs when you can uproot the tree whose seed is the 'I'-maker, deep in the heart with all its branches, fruits and leaves. Leave the mechanism of the 'I'-maker alone Kumbha says and just rest in the space in the heart."[6]

The heart, as a location of mind and body, is the dwelling place of the five kleṣas. The most deeply conditioned of the five kleṣas is asmitā, the story of self we create based on our conditioned likes and dislikes. The aim of practice is to bring duḥkha to an end by facing saṁsāra in order to uproot the egoic tendencies of the mind. Saṁsāra is literally a going around in circles. Saṁsāra is descriptive of a life of frustration where we expend a great deal of energy but live lives that keep taking us back into states of suffering.

Saṁsāra is the sense of being caught in a wheel that spins and spins, yet we can't find our way out of the cycle. When I began studying yoga postures seriously, I would practice all morning and in the afternoon I would work at a home for senior citizens. Some of the residents were quite articulate and bright, and there was a man named Walter who was especially gentle and quiet. I would sit with him under the leaded glass windows of the greenhouse, with its slate walls and mossy brick pathways, and ask him questions about Toronto and its early architecture. One day, while discussing the sad fate of some of the city's historical buildings, he made a comment about the way human and physical architecture are both subject to decay. Then he said something especially poignant: "When I think of my life as a young boy, at three or thirty, I had some of the same thoughts as when I was twelve or twenty. Now, in my late nineties, I am not sure if much has changed. I have painted and written poetry, traveled throughout Europe and made a fair amount of money. I have two grown children and I've loved my wife consistently. Despite all this I am not sure if my questions about life have been answered at all, nor if I have changed much. My neurotic self is still just as neurotic and my anxieties are exactly the same. It's as if nothing has changed."

This kind of reflection is not uncommon, and it strikes to the heart of what is meant by the term *saṁsāra*. Our psychological and physical patterns, as ingrained and self-perpetuating matrices, keep us bound to the wheel of saṁsāra, and thus the turning wheel of conditioned existence. Carl Jung often described suffering as a neurotic compulsion. He once said that "compulsion is the great mystery of human life—an involuntary motive force in the mind and body that can range all the way from mild disinterest to possession by a diabolical energy."[7] Sigmund Freud called the same activity the "compulsion to repeat," a seemingly universal tendency in the psyche to be continually caught up by something outside of awareness.[8] Twelve-step philosophy states that the "definition of insanity is repeating the same behavior and expecting different results." Most of the patterns we repeat are being repeated because they are unconscious and, by definition, outside of our awareness. Insofar as we are caught up in cycles and bundles of habit, we are stereotyped creatures, imitators and copiers of our past selves.

The teaching of karma tells us that in every moment, consciously or unconsciously, we are taking actions, however minute, that create our experience of future moments. And our actions have an effect. We put something into each moment as we dialogue with it, participate in it, and in doing so we construct the kind of experiences we have in this and future moments. If we are to grow, change, wake up, or heal in any way and to any degree, such transformation is only possible through embracing with awareness this very moment, even if it is a moment of discomfort, pain, or discontent.

So what is the path that helps us off or out of the circle? What is the path of yoga?

# 3. *Mārga*

## ESTABLISHING THE PATH

> Yoga . . . has by now become a comfortable English word, though in its more physical sense as physical or Hatha Yoga. In the Gītā, it has a wide range of meanings: path, practice, discipline, and meditation, among others. Restricting it to 'discipline' alone would be an impoverishment.
>
> —STEPHEN MITCHELL, INTRODUCTION TO THE *BHAGAVAD GĪTĀ*

YOGA AS A PATH is the way out of our present conditioning and the way toward freedom from habitually ensnaring conditions—a practice and philosophy described in widely diverse ways in texts such as the early Vedas, the *Yoga-Sutra* and the *Bhagavad Gītā.* In an Indian sense, the opposite of saṁsāra is an open space of possibility in which we can flourish and transcend where we are stuck.

Freedom only has impact if we understand it as liberation from an unfree condition. Freedom is always "freedom *from.*" Enlightenment is a movement in which we free ourselves from what obstructs and entraps us.

What constitutes the path of yoga? First, there is a sense that there is in fact a path. The Sanskrit term for "path" is *mārga,* which can refer to a trail, road, or sense of direction. The root *marg* means "to seek" or "to strive," linked also to the verbal root *mrj,* meaning "to pursue a particular direction." Likewise, a spiritual path offers us a sense of direction. A path gives us a clear trail to follow. Just as when walking in a dense forest it's hard to get around without some sort of path, in the spiritual life, we gain an intuitive sense of the path because we know intuitively when we're off the path. Even if you don't know what spiritual path you are on, you can certainly feel when you've swayed from a beneficial way.

A path also denotes that others have traveled before us. In the Aṣṭāṅga Vinyasa system of Pattabhi Jois or the method of posture sequencing taught by B.K.S. Iyengar, one finds a map of sequences that are almost identical. Their teacher, Kṛṣṇamacharya, was taught this sequence by Ramamohan Brahmacari in a cave in Tibet, and also saw diagrams of posture sequences illustrated in a now-lost text called the *Yoga Korun-tha,* reported to have been found in a library in Calcutta. Simply in terms of practice technique, a path is created by tradition and the testing out and refinement of tradition as it comes alive in the present experience of a practitioner.

Another feature of a path is that there are signs, markers, and instructions that help orient us in the landscape of the journey, a landscape often encumbered by the self-imposed ideas we create about ourselves and others. There are meditation techniques, ethics, and alignment principles that help guide us, depending on where we are within the features of the landscape, so that we can wake up to the landscape itself, only to see that landscape and practitioner are nothing other than relative categories and that the path of yoga moves beyond such categories as it ripens. Walking up a slope, or down a steep hill, or getting across a river all require different sorts of techniques. In addition, the lifestyle of a householder, a monk, a teenager, a single person, or even a man or a woman may differ, requiring different sensitivities from a teacher. When our son was born, my daily routine of three hours of early-morning āsana practice had to change. Not only did I not sleep for almost a year, there was an increased sensitivity to what others needed. Parenting became a matter of meeting necessity. If I continued to cling to my expectation of my previous form of practice, there would be suffering for myself and my family, and certainly I did not even have the stamina to practice yoga postures after many nights without sleep. It's important to have a path that is appropriate to the practitioner. A path is a mode of being in the world that is practical and accessible, yet challenges our tendency to maintain our habitual grooves of comfort. The heart always seeks a path out of discontent, but the mind and body always put up some resistance. Freud describes the path of psychotherapy in a similar way when he says that "resistance follows every step of the way."[1] However, it is equally important to remember that paying attention to what is here—the workings of the mind with its categories, judgments, and ideas about things—is the very path itself, the route and even the means.

The path of yoga is concerned with inner freedom, and there are many ways and methods of practice within the various schools of yoga. There are many different approaches to practice, sometimes even within each school, but the approach that I am distilling here has to do with freedom from the suffering inherent in saṁsāra, a practice that begins in the body, breath, and mind, and forms the basic axiom of yoga. Although there seem to be two worlds—the life of everyday chores and the disciplined dedication to formal practice—the two are not separate at all. In fact, these two sides of the yogi's life intertwine to become the very path itself, with no aspect of life separate from yoga, and yoga not separate from any thought, action, or deed. Our whole life gets rolled into practice each and every step of the way. Waking up is not an improvement of reality but rather direct contact with it.

Yoga is the practice of finding within ourselves freedom from being caught in impermanent and limited situations. In some respects we can't escape those conditions. But we can be less invested in them. Freedom is living in such a way that we are not hemmed in by, frosted with, or entangled in life's situations. We learn to preserve an inner psychological stillness of nonreactivity and ethical action, which is equivalent to freedom. Symptoms of conditioning are not only reflections of a world out of balance, but are the means by which we see the world. Jealousy is not just a manifestation of multiply determined causes but a mode of perception through which we see and eventually act. The poisons of greed, hatred, jealousy, and so on are not just symptoms that affect how we feel but on a deeper level they become, over time, the mode through which we feel. The light by which the world reflects in and through us is always modified by our conditioning, influencing not just what we perceive but how we perceive. Pattabhi Jois describes Patañjali's description of the five kleṣas as the means by which we can see how the symptoms of the heart shade and pervert our sensual experience of day-to-day living in mind and body.

Enlightenment (*mokṣa*) is here and now. It occurs when we free ourselves from ego clinging and become more transparent, letting go of the armoring, carapace, or protection that we think of as ourselves, dissolving any separation with the greater world. This means opening up to our own suffering as well as to the discontent in the world around us. At that point, our spiritual practice rises to the level of asking, How can I be so concerned with my own spiritual practice when there is so much suffering in the world? How can we live a life that can optimally benefit others? The long point of the opus of this process is seeing the self out of balance in a world out of balance, so that we practice to harmonize both, because they are not, as we once thought, separate from each other. Through removing the centrality of "me," we open up to the world at large so that internal and external, inner and outer, me and you, become conceptual designations only, not the reality of felt experience, which is not two but one.

The path of yoga helps us find an authentic and meaningful response to having been born and ultimately having to die. Opening up to this truth can be terrifying; it can also open us up to the amazing promise that yoga offers: freedom from trying to create permanence in an ever-changing existence. Although our core beliefs make us feel secure and somewhat unchanging, yoga practice opens us to the reality of being an ever-changing flow of conditions arising and passing away, and completely empty of any trace of permanence except for the truth of relational existence. The basis of everything is boundless.

Beginning with body, mind, and breath as they are experienced in the present moment, yoga practice deals with the common hypnotic state of suffering and a conditioned existence in which we find ourselves spinning. This unconsciousness has, as a result, chronic physical and psychological holding patterns. Once we begin to see the way our conditions are constructed, we begin taking them apart until the very last conditional pattern is revealed: clinging to the notions of "I, me, and mine." In finding freedom from the captive consequences of "me" and "mine," we no longer experience reality as an isolated self. Then we become not only better able to relate to our conditioned existence, but more engaged in the interconnected world of relationships and thus the complex and heartfelt domain of action, compassion, and ethical responsibility.

# 4. Embodying the Path

The one light appears in diverse forms.

—*Atharva-Veda*

For yoga to continue as a living tradition, it is important to study, practice, and continually wrestle with the basic teachings offered by teachers and texts. Without committed practice and critical engagement with the tradition of yoga, yoga becomes a tradition of only antiquarian interest. The poet Czeslaw Milosz writes, "What good is poetry if it cannot save nations or people?"[1] Can we not ask the same of yoga?

When we take ideas taught within the yoga traditions as ultimate truths, yoga becomes dogmatic and oppressive. Then there is always a practitioner, like Rama in the *Yoga Vāsiṣṭa* or Arjuna in the *Bhagavad Gītā,* who asks, "What do these elite practices have to do with my suffering and my life in the face of death? What is this life that I find myself in?" For the student who approaches practice and teachings with an open and critical mind, practice and awakening become less to do with ideological or orthodox understanding and more to do with a response in the here and now to the great questions of life. Yoga is not about conforming to other people's definitions of practice but simply an authentic response to the questions presented by our life, our path. If yoga points at the truth of existence, that very existence must be available to us in every moment, not as a new belief system or a utopia to arrive at in a future life, but something we can touch, maintain, and discover for ourselves.

"Better to do one's own work dutifully than to do another's well," Kṛṣṇa says to Arjuna in the final chapter of the *Bhagavad Gītā*. One of the last teachings on yoga in the epic of the *Bhagavad Gītā,* much like the initial teachings of *abhyāsa* (practice) and *vairāgya* (letting go) in the *Yoga-Sutra,* is to continually test out the field between theory and practice.[2] Otherwise, we are practicing someone else's ideas or the teachings from another culture without genuinely wresting with those ideas ourselves. For yoga to be a living tradition, we need to integrate committed practice with a teacher alongside critical engagement with the core axioms of the particular yoga system we are studying so that the teachings come alive in this culture, in this time, in this human experience. The poet Jorge Luis Borges writes,

> Everything happens for the first time,
> But in that way it is eternal.
> Whoever lights a match in the dark is inventing fire.
> Whoever goes down to a river goes down to the Ganges.
> Whoever reads my words is inventing them.[3]

Yoga is timeless. This does not mean it is eternal or ephemeral, but simply available, always, in each unfolding moment, when we settle into the essence of who we are. The great questions of life and death are settled in the stillness of the mind and the direct actions of a self unfettered by itself. A seeming paradox at first, the yoga practitioner is nothing other than the vast range of the universe. The Ganges becomes the central axis of one's own body, and the essence of the body is discovered to be nothing other than the great rivers of the earth, the vast sky, and the winds of the breath. We practice in whatever conditions we find ourselves: depressed, flowing, polluted, clear, transparent, slow, or thick as mud.

## *Lowering Your Center of Gravity*

The practice of yoga postures, what is commonly referred to as Hatha Yoga, belongs within the domain of Tantra Yoga. The term *tantra* is a combination of two roots: *tan* (to loom, warp, or do something in precise detail) and *tra* (to protect). Tantra begins with noticing the breath and its energetic aspects in the center of the body in great detail. What at first seems like the obvious rhythm of the breath, for example, opens up to show us the subtle winds that make up the breath, the impermanent nature of all of our thoughts and feelings, and the inherent nonseparation between the breath and the great vibration that is all living reality. This precision of attention interrupts our common mental distractions, the root causes of duḥkha.

While there are many misconceptions about tantra as a sexual practice or an esoteric model of visualization, and while some forms of tantra do include such practices, the wider sense of tantra is the study of the energetic relationship of mind and body in order to shift the mind out of its distracted habits into a deeper relationship with the basic constituents of nature. As we begin working with mind and body, we become acutely aware of energetic shifts in the body—feelings, temperature, nervous system, breathing. Learning how to work with the energies of mind and body is the core practice of tantra. Tantra is psychological in essence because we have to learn to let go of the momentum of distracted and reactive mental habits in order to feel and move with energetic changes in the body. The body is studied and felt, sculpted and investigated, until it becomes treated as a microcosm of the greater universe. The study of reality begins with the body because there is no perceived world independent of mind and body.

In Hatha Yoga, the center of the body is the base of the pelvic diaphragm. Like a wheel (*chakra*) or circle, the pelvic diaphragm floats above and is stretched between the dense corners of the pelvis: two sitting bones, the pubic bone, and the coccyx. Like looking down inside the base of a flower pot, the internal symmetry of the pelvic floor is circular with an empty center hollowed above the perineum. At the end of an exhale, a contraction occurs behind the abdominal well that ends in the center of the pelvic floor. This is called *mūla bandha* (the rooting bond), in which the breath creates tone in the pelvic floor and the mind is present enough to experience the action. There are two key points here: (1) that the breath cycle is organized to complete the exhale in its entirety, and (2) that one's awareness is focused and steady enough to be present at the end of the out-breath. This is but one example of the yoking of mind, breath, and body. Tantra is the science of paying attention, and the basic practices of attention begin in the body via the breath. Like many yoga practices, physical technique and psychology cannot be separated.

The center of the pelvic floor is also the center of gravity for a human being. In yoga we are always moving toward the center of things: thoughts, feelings, sensations, breath cycles. All movement is initiated from the center of the pelvic floor, and the breath as an energetic pattern completes itself in a pause at mūla bandha and begins again where it ends. The death and rebirth of the breath cycle in physical form is felt most acutely in the pelvic diaphragm as we come in direct contact with the arising, spreading, and eventual contraction and disbanding of each movement as felt in the stream of each breath. We pay attention to the pelvic diaphragm in breathing practices and yoga postures not only because it challenges our ability to stay present with one simple thing, but because it's the center of the human body, and a microcosmic window into the center of reality.

In the center of the human body we find the center of all things because when breath, mind, and body come together in an instant of experience, reality unfolds. Reality unfolds when the mind can stay completely present in a breath cycle, especially at the completion of an exhale. The exhale completes itself in the pelvic floor, the center of gravity, the resting place of the mind. The *Chandogya Upaniṣad* describes this clearly:

> Just as a bird tied by a string, after flying in various directions without finding a resting-place elsewhere settles down (at last) at the place where it is bound, so also the mind, my dear, after flying in various directions without finding a resting-place elsewhere, settles down in breath, for the mind, my dear, is bound to breath.[4]

Yoga psychology sees the mind and breath as bound together in the frame of the human body. There is no mind without breath, no stillness in body without stillness in mind, and no stillness in the mind without a breath that has settled.

Mūla bandha, much like yoga itself, is not something you do but rather something that occurs spontaneously when you are present with the completion of an exhalation. When the breath naturally comes to completion, there is a feeling of toning and drawing up in the center of the pelvic region just above the perineum. Once the pelvic diaphragm tones, as the out-breath turns around and becomes an in-breath, the center of the floor curls up and lifts toward the roof of the mouth, turning from a concave into a convex apex. This was discovered by yogis as a perfect object of meditation because it requires concentration, excellent breathing, steadiness in the nerves, patience, and interest in the body and mind in this very moment, and the same truth can be discovered by all of us when we focus our attention in one place for long enough. Mūla bandha is a spontaneous gesture in the center of the human body that occurs when the breath cycle is allowed to complete itself without the interference of the mind. Hatha Yoga is the cultivation of careful and precise observation via imagination and feeling, and forms the basis of later psychological techniques in meditation practice. Treating our yoga postures and breathing practices as meditation technique opens up deeper and deeper feeling pathways, and it is through those very pathways that the world moves through us.

We pay attention, even when nothing is happening. "If something is boring after two minutes, try it for four," writes the composer John Cage. "If still boring, then eight. Then sixteen. Then thirty-two. Eventually one discovers that it is not boring at all."[5] Mūla bandha is a meditation technique that uses the energetic movements in the body, via the breath cycle, as a neutral anchor point for the mind.

As we slow down and investigate our experience from moment to moment, we are, in essence, studying the way we organize and construct our experience. Slowing down gives us an opportunity to get to know what it is we are investigating, rather than the usual tendency of superimposing our theories on whatever it is we see. Learning the techniques of mūla bandha teaches us to be present with the feelings, thoughts, emotions, and breath cycles occurring right in the center of human experience.

The root teacher in yoga is always the present moment. The word *guru* comes over to English as "gravity." *Guru* denotes a center of gravity. The root *gu* stands for darkness; *ru* for its removal. The guru, or the teacher, is one who sheds light in the darkness of avidyā. The guru is one who understands the law of gravity and other basic laws of the universe, including the law of impermanence and the truth of duḥkha. The guru, although sometimes embodied in an external person or entity, is actually your own center of gravity. The manifestation of these teachings is ultimately experienced within one's own body and mind so that the heart opens up, revealing an internal center of gravity. Connecting with one's center of gravity is the embodiment of stillness.

One of the most radical axioms of yoga is that the factors at work in and the elements that make up the universe at large are the same as those at work in each individual mind as it organizes experience. Watching the breath reverse its course at the bottom of an exhalation cuts into the center of reality itself if our attention is totally focused. "What's here is everywhere," says the narrator of the epic *Mahābhārata,* "and what isn't here is nowhere."[6] The way we process the sensory data that arrive through the sense organs and the mind demonstrates how we organize our experience of the cosmos. Watching the breath can be like watching the birth-and-death cycle of the universe. It's all right here in this immediate moment of perception, organization, and experience.

Why this is significant for our practice is that since we construct our experience from moment to moment, we also construct our suffering. Our experience of suffering or dissatisfaction (duḥkha) always occurs in the present moment. So we don't leave the present moment in order to work with suffering; rather, we focus directly on the processing of present experience because that is where the crucial troubles play themselves out most clearly. We stop looking outside of ourselves for the causes of suffering and waiting in vain for the world to change so that we can finally feel peace. Instead, duḥkha is seen to be nothing other than present reality multiplied by resistance.

We don't necessarily look to the past for explanations or worry about repeating addictive patterns in the future. The past is encoded in the present. Therefore we stay with what is arising right now and investigate it without coming out of it. If yoga denotes union, then yoga is the cultivation of no-separation, where we can be in something with clarity without separating from it. Described in another way, there is nothing to cultivate because underneath distraction and aversion, everything is already joined.

Right here and right now is where everything important is happening. This is where we pay attention. The breath and the body are always present, so we breathe our circumstances. Then we develop the skills necessary to deal with difficulty rather than reinforcing patterns of aversion. This helps us use the mind efficiently—as a locator of the proper frame of reference. The proper qualities of mind are needed to see something clearly, to feel what is there to be felt and allow it to pass on. Then we gain wisdom. The ability to separate the act from its object helps us become more sensitive to the act before it becomes overwhelming. When we can observe the coming and going of chronic pain, for example, we can learn how to be in it, how to bear it, how to breathe with it as it arises and passes a way. This is a powerful skill. This is the skill of being able to see something arising as it arises, change as it changes, and pass away as it does, without being caught up in it.

In chronic or any other kind of pain, including emotional pain, sometimes we spend so much effort trying to get away from it that we actually increase it. We feel pain in the body and then react to that pain with aversion, stories of likes and dislikes, memory, association, and conceptualization. This cycle happens so fast that it is almost impossible to see. Yoga slows down the way we perceive our experience so that we can see how we organize it. If there is a moment of suffering or a moment of joy, we can see how we put those moments together.

## *Participating in Each Moment*

When we continually run away from our experience, we plant seeds of repetition: the next time the same experience occurs, we will meet that experience with the conditioned response systems we have constructed and reinforced in mind, body, and nervous system. We create a feedback loops in the *saṁskāras* (psychophysical grooves) and in the *nadis* (feeling and feedback pathways) that keep us running away from the pain. Or, could it be possible that we could notice pain when it arises and ride it out to its dissolution? In this way, one eventually becomes so familiar with the patterns underlying their occurrence that one can get under them before they take over. Eventually we eliminate all forms of reaction. When there is no reaction, we are free to take action. In other words, when reactive patterns are suspended or let go of altogether, we can respond in any given situation without reaction to that situation. Reaction and response are not the same. Why? "Response" refers to a spontaneous way of being in which we can accept and recognize what is actually occurring and take an appropriate action. Since we are usually so reactive, it is hard to first recognize what is actually occurring. Our perception is clouded with preference. Once we can recognize what is happening in a moment of experience, we can accept it, allowing it to unfold without trying to get away from it. When we can accept something, we can investigate it in depth and release our instinctive movements toward identifying with the content of experience. Then pain is pain, a feeling is a feeling—all aspects of nature, coming, transforming, and passing on.

In the course of paying close attention to the breath, mind, and body, we discover that the experience of the present moment consists of results from past actions and present actions. This is the law of karma: that volitional action always has an effect. Previous experience influences present experience, and what we do in the present influences the way we experience the future. This means that karma operates in feedback loops. The present moment is shaped by both past and present actions. Present action shapes not only the future but also the present. There is nothing that separates who we are from all that comes to be. Our actions and intentions all contribute to how things are. In short, our dispositions are implicated in everything we do. Our experience is always filtered through our preconditioned sense organs and mind. So we are like filters, unique and unrepeatable synthesizers. Thus our work is to filter our experience in a way that does not negatively contribute to the activity of the world.

The way we experience the present moment is participatory. Our actions have consequences. Usually *karma* is translated into English as "fate." But this is a misunderstanding. The word *vipāka* refers to the effect of an action. The word *karma,* however, refers to both volitional action and its effects. "Wherever there is fire," Kṛṣṇa says in the *Bhagavad Gītā,* "there is smoke."[7] Our actions are always followed by residue.

There is no-thing that exists independent of our intentions and actions, no substance, no answer, no final separation between who we are and the deep questions life presents us. Causality in terms of yoga means that when see inordinate degrees of suffering and greed, envy and fear, aggression and inflexibility in the world around us, and when we also see that those are qualities we don't want to contribute to the culture, then our practice of mind, heart, and body becomes a practice of filtering those potentials in all of us. I must meditate on causality so that I can work with my own capacity for greed, violence, or intolerance, and as such my whole being becomes a filter for the culture. It is as though by practicing what at first seems like an internal practice, it becomes a form of social action. Causality allows us to see that our internal work of meditation flows out into the world around us depending on the way we participate in each moment. When we understand causality—the way we participate in each moment—we begin to see the yoga of relationship: we cannot seek truth or change outside of ourselves. No matter what aspect of the path calls you, the commitment in this practice is to waking up, not doctrine, or theology, or self-improvement. Any reduction in suffering is worthwhile, even if it's simply coming to a yoga class and feeling our way into stillness or becoming aware perhaps just once in the day of our breathing.

The practice of noticing the difference between pure awareness (*puruṣa*) and the fluctuating objects of consciousness is about allowing space in the heart, in the mind, in the body so that we depart from habitual mental constructs and psychological delusions, not from thinking altogether but from conceiving in conceited and predisposed ways. Awakening is the ongoing process of lifting the veils in the mind that divide things into opposites, and thus enlightenment is becoming who we really are, free to take action without feeling as though "my" actions benefit the other. Through taking wholesome action and understanding the habits that inform unwholesome action we decondition the heart into such a natural state of openness that we see no existence in the universe as separate from this very self. Yoga works against our most problematic duality: taking actions in the belief that we are truly separate from the world. Habits dying and a self predisposed to what is greater than self go hand in hand, arm in arm. Without the passing away of habit, the yoked nature of the present moment remains concealed. Irvin Yalom makes the point in psychological language:

> To live in the present above time is to have no future, and to have no future is to accept death—yet this man cannot do. He cannot accept death and therefore neither can he live in the Now; and not living in the Now, he lives not at all.[8]

"Death" in this case is the death of habit—the ongoing letting go of the thoughts that keep us "concealed and wrapped" in our self-centered versions of reality. Any creation of a separate self is a defense against letting go, and gives rise to the six poisons of duḥkha, the six enemies in the heart.

# 5. The Eight Limbs

We Western practitioners (I cannot speak for non-Western practitioners) have come to realize, somewhat reluctantly, that our spiritual practice has not eliminated some of our basic psychological ills, including deep anxieties, fears, and neuroses. This is hard to admit. We came to practice, and continue to practice, because we believe in the liberative freedom promised by texts, teachers, and practices. But as time moves forward, we see that practice sometimes leaves many stones unturned. How is it that we can develop strong and flexible posture practices, deep states of meditation, or advanced prāṇāyāma techniques, yet still leave many of our deep-seated habits and thoughts untouched?

Many practitioners report that periods of deep practice can sometimes be followed by periods of confusion, depression, or anxiety. Returning from workshops or retreats, practitioners have to face the reality of relational existence. For most of us, it is the world of relationship that brings up our deepest holding patterns. That being so, it is the clarifying work of attending to the push of habit and the pull of relationship that forms the first limb of yoga practice.

Without beginning on the first limb of the path, the *yamas* (restraints), our practice may bypass important developmental activities crucial to our psychological growth, including cultivating relationships with diverse people and learning how to navigate relational existence in general. Sincere and eccentric relationships demand of us authenticity and present-centeredness. Virginia Woolf described this succinctly in a diary entry of June 22, 1940: "More to the point and less composed."[1]

As our yoga practice matures, we find ourselves less accompanied by self-reference and, in place of self-interest, a new kind of movement in tune with the world. The practice of waking up the mind and body and the practice of stilling mind and body go hand in hand in what is referred to as the royal (*rāja*) path of yoga, described by Patañjali as the eight-limbed path. This path, known as Aṣṭāṅga yoga (*aṣ*—"eight," *tāṇga*—"limbs"), involves the simultaneous practice of eight limbs, or branches.

The poisons Pattabhi Jois referred to prior to teaching about the kleṣas have as their common denominator self-centeredness. Envy, anger, jealousy, greed, and scattered desire all resolve to fortify our sense of self with an unsatisfying and ultimately untenable solution. The yamas keep these diverse and conflicting impulses in check. Desire, for example, is necessary for anyone who pursues a spiritual path, but it's the act of seeing through desire by holding it in check that ultimately transforms our relation to it and to others. Without a practice that increases the clarity of thought, perception, and feeling, we wind up moving through the world enclosed in a soliloquy that leaves in its wake alienation, harm, and dissatisfaction. We have a moral obligation to the entire ecological web of existence to wake up from self-pity and self-promotion in order to attend to our place in the world with sensitivity and wisdom.

The eight limbs are as follows:

1. *Yama*s (external restraints): the clarification of one's relationship to the world of people and objects. There are five practices associated with this limb:

    *Ahiṁsā* (not harming, nonviolence)
    *Satya* (honesty, being truthful)
    *Asteya* (not taking what is not freely given, not stealing)
    *Brahmacharya* (wise use of energy, including sexual energy)
    *Aparigraha* (not being acquisitive, not accumulating what is not essential)

2. *Niyamas* (internal restraints): personal principles governing the cultivation of insight.
   *Śauca* (purification)
   *Santoṣa* (contentment)
   *Tapas* (discipline, patience)
   *Svādhyāya* (self-study, contemplation)
   *Īśvara-pranidhāna* (devotion, dedication to the ideal of pure awareness)
3. *Āsana* (posture): cultivation of profound physical and psychological steadiness and ease in mind, breath, and body.
4. *Prāṇāyāma* (breath and energetic regulation): sustained observation and relaxation of all aspects of breathing, bringing about a natural refinement of the mind-body process through the stilling of the respiratory process.
5. *Pratyāhāra* (withdrawing of the senses): a naturally occurring uncoupling of sense organs and sense objects as awareness interiorizes.
6. *Dhāraṇā* (concentration meditation): locking awareness on a single object (such as sound, breath, sensations in the body) until the field of awareness becomes singular and focused.
7. *Dhyāna* (absorption): concentration deepens to the point where subject and object dissolve.
8. *Samādhi* (integration): the sustained experience of concentration, in which there is a complete integration of subject and object, revealing pure awareness as the nondual substratum of reality; no-separation.

Some teachers describe the first four limbs as external and the last four limbs as internal. Others say that you practice the first four limbs with sheer will and then the last four limbs occur spontaneously. However, this is not the traditional approach to the eight limbs, nor what Patañjali intended. A balanced practice is the simultaneous investigation of all eight limbs as each limb compliments every other limb. Richard Freeman describes the eight limbs as a complete yoga practice,

> . . . which is evolving into deep and spontaneous meditation and complete liberation. The variety of limbs guarantees that the awareness operates in all spheres of one's life, so that no distortion, perversion or fantasy will attempt to usurp the solid ground of real Yogic insight. In many of the yoga Upaniṣads the eight limbs are further expanded into fifteen. The advantage of considering the path of yoga to have many aspects is that one is encouraged not to neglect the moral, the ethical, the interpersonal, the physiological, the esoteric and the meditative aspects of practice. The term Aṣṭāṅga implies both simultaneous realization of all these interrelated aspects of practice and a logical step-by-step progression where one limb prepares one to truly practice the next one.[2]

In contemporary yoga practices we often jump into the third limb, of āsana, and end up with a fragmented and imbalanced yoga practice because it has no roots. The rooting of a practice occurs when one starts at the beginning with the ethical codes that Patañjali outlines as the stepping-stone to further practices.

The root problems in our world—violence, greed, anger, inflexibility, intolerance—are at core a problem of perception and consciousness. In terms of perception, our attitudes, behaviors, and actions are conditioned in ways that are not challenged within culture. And in terms of consciousness, there seems to be a fundamental existential dislocation, one that has both cognitive and ethical dimensions. That is, individual and collective duḥkha both stem from a disorientation in our understanding of reality, and a distortion of what we are actually experiencing. Because our root problems have to do with perception and consciousness, this means that any viable solution must be framed in terms of a transformation of consciousness. It requires an attempt to arrive at a more accurate grasp of the human situation in its full depth and breadth, and a turning of the mind and heart in a new direction, a direction commensurate with the new understanding, one that brings light and peace rather than strife and distress. This begins with the cultivation of a practice rooted in human and ecological relationship rather than individual success or achievement. Yoga is a practice of horizontal transcendence (you and me in relation to each other) rather than vertical transcendence (my practice for my own freedom).

Many practitioners of Hatha Yoga have a partial view of practice since the cornerstone of the path, the yamas, is bypassed or avoided altogether. The foundation of the spiritual path of yoga is ethics. Ethics forms the foundation of yoga practice, because as a set of suggestions for how to live, it goes right to the heart of our actions of body, speech, and mind. The ethical principles of nonharming, truthfulness, the wise use of sexual energy, not stealing, and nonacquisitiveness refer to the honest examination and transformation of our physical actions and interpersonal relations. They not only apply to the way we act in external relationships, they also apply to our internal states as well. We apply these ethical principles to all relationships, including intrapsychic.

If our yoga practice went no further than the first limb—ethics-based restraints—we would still experience great benefit, as would those around us. Ethical principles keep us kind, sensitive, and balanced in our internal states as well as in our response to the external; the yamas place us over and again squarely in community, even in the community of characters and energies that move through our internal awareness. They keep us grounded in the world of relationship, which includes other people, animals, the environment, the elements, and even one's internal states of mind and body.

The yamas also help keep the mind and the energetic flow of the body from being scattered. They help us maintain our equilibrium while being in and of the world. This also helps us study our own psychology, since we watch closely our intentions when taking any given action. Having the yamas as guides allows us to see clearly the nature of our intentions so that we can monitor our volitional actions and engage appropriately with whatever circumstance we find ourselves in. The yamas remind us that the purpose of yoga is to show how experience can be made a source of creative action. In fact sometimes the most negative characteristics of one's personality are more prominent sources of wisdom than the positive aspects, because they are the details and encumbrances that we've struggled with most, know most intimately, and have learned how to wrestle, restrain, and transform.

In addition to teaching yoga I also have a psychotherapy practice. In my continual training as a psychotherapist I am always amazed at how strict the guidelines are about professional ethics, such as maintaining confidentiality or not having inappropriate sexual relations with our patients—yet the psychology of ethics on a personal level are never discussed. One of the greatest differences between the Western and the yogic models of psychology and psychological methods of transformation is that yoga begins with a very clear articulation and description of ethics, while Western psychology avoids altogether the topic of ethical action except in terms of professional conduct. It is surprising that the training for people in the helping professions, especially since they tend to be the people who help us make decisions and take action, does not include training in the psychology of being ethical. Personal commitment to the yamas helps us work with our deeply conditioned and seemingly instinctual patterns of reactivity so that our intentions and actions can be motivated by clarity of mind and generosity rather than chronic patterns of reactivity or self-interest.

When we move farther along the path of yoga, much like hiking up a mountain, we want to travel lightly. This means not bringing along the weighty baggage of inappropriate relationships, guilt, shame, and the manifestations of a mind caught in greed, hatred, or delusion.

Unlinking actions of body, speech, and mind leave in their wake difficulty and stress. Traveling lightly begins in the first limb through the purification of our relationships both internally and externally. The demands of desire are endless. Like insatiable energies, they continually strive for satisfaction by creating in the mind the belief that something outside of ourselves can last eternally. The entire path of yoga, from beginning to end, orients the practitioner toward a life of renunciation. What is most difficult to renounce, however, is the desire for a solid and permanent sense of self. The yamas, as a cornerstone of practice, keeps the practitioner embedded in the world of relationships in order to use this relational matrix as a means of seeing through a self-centered reality. The yamas safeguard against the tendency to act out habitual patterns of reactivity.

# 6. Practicing the *Yamas*

WE FUNNEL all ethical codes or precepts through three modes of practice: body, speech, and mind. We practice *ahiṁsā* (nonviolence) with regard to body, speech, and mind. We practice nonviolence in regard to our own body and to the bodies of others. Then we practice nonharming in how we speak to ourselves about ourselves and also how we speak to others. Of course nonviolence of speech also connotes the ability to listen. Speaking and listening go together. Then we practice nonharming in our own mind and also refrain from harmful thoughts about others. It's always easier to critique the world than it is to see how we have and are contributing to the momentum of violence and inflexibility that we so easily see outside of ourselves. Negative gossip, not kind and thoughtful reflection, sells newspapers.

I was once in an elevator in downtown Toronto with a five-year-old boy. We were both fascinated by the recent developments in elevator technology in which instead of pressing a button to take us to the floor of our destination we were asked to simply say "Floor Thirty-three" out loud and a computer would signal the elevator to take us to the appropriate floor.

Realizing this computer was impersonal, the five-year-old started blurting out all kinds of things. "Stupid elevator" turned into every other form of slang he could muster until, after he'd repeatedly sworn at this computer, we finally arrived at our floor. I turned to him and asked, "How does that feel? How does it feel saying all those things to a computer?"

"Not so good," he replied. Then we stepped off the elevator. He was quiet for the next few minutes.

Sometimes, thinking negative thoughts, though they may not directly affect others, has a negative effect on our own felt sense of being. Where do my actions end? Do my intentions ripple through the world? Do my actions come back to me, and if so, how? Isn't my self-realization your self-realization and vice versa?

Establishing a solid basis in nonharming, both internally and externally, roots our yoga practice in an understanding of karma. Karma refers to volitional action and its effects. Every action we take has an effect. Here is an example of how Patañjali uses the notion of karma in his description of ethical conduct with regard to nonharming in body, speech, and mind:

> 2.33 Unwholesome thoughts can be neutralized by cultivating wholesome ones.
>
> 2.34 We ourselves may act upon unwholesome thoughts, such as wanting to harm someone, or we may cause or condone them in others; unwholesome thoughts may arise from greed, anger or delusion; they may be mild, moderate or extreme; but they never cease to ripen into ignorance and suffering. This is why one must cultivate wholesome thoughts.
>
> 2.35 Being firmly grounded in nonviolence creates an atmosphere in which others can let go of their hostility.[1]

These passages not only show the interrelation of our actions and our psychological conditioning, they orient the yoga practitioner to contemplate and take action in the world of relationship. Notice in Patañjali's description of nonviolence how he is always balancing his teachings between the internal world of the practitioner and the external world as well. Patañjali does not describe the result of a nonharmful attitude in terms of one's personal practice; instead he suggests that when one is firmly grounded in nonviolence, it affects others so that they may drop their defensive strategies and hostility. Otherwise, it's like a nuclear superpower telling all other countries that they cannot have nuclear weapons. The premise of nonviolence in this context is that it takes two to maintain a relationship of violence. Nonviolent relationship needs to be initiated by a firm commitment to being honest about the effect of one's choices and actions. Therefore, we begin by acting with less harmful intentions, cultivating an atmosphere in which others can do the same.

Nonviolence of speech means that our speech should be honest and loving even when direct and strong. Oftentimes, compassion is illustrated in Indian art as a sharp sword that cuts through delusion. The *vajra* (thunderbolt) symbolizes the way in which clear, compassionate action cuts through indecisiveness or dishonesty. Since words cause both joy and discontent, we meditate on our actions of speech continually so that we do not speak untruthfully, gossip, exaggerate, or try to impress others. This also means using our words clearly to speak up for those who cannot do so themselves, and using our voice to bring awareness to forms of injustice, even if speaking out means threatening our own safety or security. An action based on self-image is never an honest or unrehearsed gesture. There is no self-image, we begin to see, without suffering. "Human beings," the philosopher Hilary Putnam writes, "are self-surprising creatures." We may surprise ourselves with our inherent honesty and kindness when we make a commitment to the yamas as wise possibilities for ethical engagement in everyday life.

Treated as dogmatic codes, the yamas become limiting and rigid. Being free of self-image through the honest practice of letting go and a deep commitment to others through following through on the yamas opens up room for spontaneity and responsiveness. Who knows what letting go will bring? The yamas are not codes or commandments but simply suggestions that honor the way a wise person lives. One does not get into trouble for breaking a code but rather studies their experience and the effects of their actions. Yoga is about bringing awareness to our actions of body, speech, and mind.

When people come to our center to study yoga, especially when we have time to meet one-on-one, we always begin by teaching the first yama. Teaching about nonharming immediately sets students thinking about their practice as both internal and external, which early on cuts off the tendency to create distinction between formal and informal practice. Also, beginning with teaching about nonharming helps students relate to their experience without judgment or the negative superimposition of poor self-esteem. Instead of negatively judging our habitual patterns, we can get to know ourselves with an awareness free of limiting self-judgment.

After a student is grounded in the principle of ahiṁsā, we move slowly through each limb, practicing every stage of every limb. Without the underpinning of ethics, practice is separate from the relational world. When the various egoic and inflexible conditions are seen for what they are and eventually transformed, one is capable of much greater intimacy and a fuller involvement with every aspect of experience. Otherwise one can practice great yoga postures while their inner psychological world goes untouched. We can do wonderful arm balances, but our relationships are a mess; or we can teach yoga postures but have no insight, compassion, or wisdom. Seeing clearly means that we tune the mind-body process in order to see how we are not separate from all beings and all things, and thus the practice and sharing of yoga is a means of liberating the personality from self-reference, numbness, and existential paralysis.

## Satya *and* Asteya

After ahiṁsā, one contemplates satya (honesty of body, speech, and mind). This includes being honest with ourselves about our bodies (i.e., self-image), being honest in how we speak with others, and also being honest in our thoughts. From there we practice *asteya* (not stealing). We can translate "not stealing" very specifically, as in not stealing from stores or others, where we can cause harm directly or indirectly. All of the yamas are intertwined in sequential order and loop back into one another, in the same way that the layers of the body warp and weave in an interdependent matrix. The common link in the chain of the yamas is meditating on karma and taking actions rooted in nonharming. Nonviolence makes the repercussions of not being honest plainly obvious, because being dishonest causes harm. The same is true for nonstealing. When we steal, not only are we being dishonest, we are causing violence. The actions of violence, dishonesty, and stealing all arise from three sources, according to Patañjali: "greed, ill will or delusion." But, as stated earlier in Patañjali's description of nonharming, ". . . they never cease to ripen into ignorance and suffering." In other words, beginning from the first limb, we see how yoga begins with a fundamental shift in one's behavior, attitude, and relations through a shift in one's psychology. The psychology of stealing, as an example, is a product of an unsatisfied mind. Nonstealing is inextricably linked with one's desires, writes Gandhi:

> We are not always aware of our real needs, and most of us improperly multiply our wants, and thus unconsciously make thieves out of ourselves. If we devote some thought to the subject, we shall find that we can get rid of a number of our wants. One who follows the observance of non-stealing will bring a progressive reduction of his own wants. Much of the distressing poverty of this world has arisen out of the breaches of the principle of non-stealing.[3]

We can also practice asteya in subtle ways. *Asteya* literally means "not taking what is not freely given." As a practice, nonstealing, like all of the other yamas, orients us toward the transparency of all things and their interrelationship. Oftentimes we steal space by taking up more space than we need, physically and psychically. When we are impatient, we are wrestling with time, caught in a relationship of friction, which is why impatience is considered stealing time. J. Krishnamurti says that "patience is not of time."[4] When we are patient, we are not aware of the time, so when there is impatience, there is an acute awareness of time. Sometimes an hour feels like a minute and sometimes a minute feels like a day.

## Brahmacharya

*Brahmacharya* for the monk means celibacy while for the householder it refers to the wise use of energy, especially sexual. Insatiable desire not only intoxicates us but turns others into objects. Nonharming as it applies in the sexual domain of body, speech, and mind becomes brahmacharya. This includes much more than not having sex that harms others, because it includes balancing sexual energy within one's own body, in speech, and also in mind. Sexual fantasies constantly turn others into objects of our desire and in so doing prevent a true meeting of another. Aside from the energetic distraction of sexual fantasy, it is important to notice how fantasy often serves the egoic function of the mind rather than the heart.

This is not so to say sex or the topic of sexuality is off-limits, because both must be embraced as sacred and keys to our psychological maturing. To turn a blind eye to matters of sexuality will always lead to repression. If we try to push away our sexual energy, we end up with a fragmented consciousness that cannot sustain impermanent and natural patterns of energy. As has been well reported, the avoidance or repression of sexual energy in monastic communities, where no one dares to talk about the reality of sexual energy in contemporary life, leads to the underground acting out of those very same energies. Without attachment or aversion, we investigate our circumstances, whatever they are. So instead of pushing sexual energy underground, we work with sexual energy as it arises and passes away, and experience the energy simply as energy: impermanent and not "me" or "mine."

When we depersonalize sexual energy, it has less of an intoxicating or magnetic effect and then we can work with it in a way that is wise. Brahmacharya is not an ethical code based on fear or prudery but rather one that encourages an honest appraisal of the energies that move within us, their effects, and how to work with the movements of energy, sexual or otherwise. When we bring awareness to the way that any form of sexual relation motivated by craving cannot dissipate the feelings of loneliness or longing that we are trying to satisfy but actually creates more suffering, frustration, and isolation, we become determined not to engage in sexual relations without mutual understanding, love, and commitment. In sexual relations, writes Thich Nhat Hanh, "it is important to be aware of future suffering that may be caused by our actions of body, speech, or mind. We come to know that to preserve the happiness of ourselves and others, we must respect the rights and commitments of ourselves and others."[5]

Sexual energy tempered by the yamas means treating our bodies with respect and preserving our energy for the realization of our practice ideals, which are compassion and no-separation. This means being as aware as possible of the effect of bringing new life into the world and also, as Thich Nhat Hanh encourages, "meditating deeply on the world into which we are bringing life."[6] Even in sexual relations where there is not a literal new life-form being created (i.e., an infant), we can meditate on the way in which every sexual encounter creates a new life of relations between two people. New cultures begin with two. Our yoga community has several practitioners who are same-sex partners without children yet who return often to the teachings of brahmacharya to remind themselves how every encounter between people, especially sexual encounters, creates a new kind of relationship, a new form of life. Brahmacharya as a guideline is wide enough to include all people and types of relationships without regard for one's sexual orientation.

## Aparigraha

*Aparigraha* (nonacquisitiveness), comes from the root *grah,* which means "to grasp." Georg Feuerstein translates *aparigraha* as "greedlessness."[7] While this is an excellent translation, it is important to capture the fact that this is not the practice of greedlessness as a final end point, because that might be more idealistic than realistic, but the practice of not acquiring based on greed. Like the other yamas, karma comes down to intention. Again, this is not something one is punished for, but simply a guideline for a wise way to live that promotes psychological stillness and the transformation of self-centered desire. Owning things or accumulating knowledge adds nothing to a life authentically lived. Again, these restraints are designed to restrain the momentum of our self-centered position in the scale of perception and instead turn us toward making the daring leap of changing our habitually exploitative ways.

# 7. The *Yamas* Beyond Dualism

ATTEMPTING TO PRACTICE ideals like brahmacharya in daily life is challenging, but like all the yamas, such ideals encourage transformation by which the alienation between myself and the world ultimately diminishes and a sense of mutual connection, responsibility, and empathy progressively matures. This is the actualization of nonduality. A lack of self-preoccupation allows us to be devoted to the welfare of others.

Free from the stress of dualistic fixation, and the ongoing habit of dividing the relational field into two—a subject and an object for the subject—we emerge free and better able to respond to others. In any form of fantasy or fixation there is no immediate and direct contact with the other. The other becomes an object that we steal for our sensual or imaginative gratification. This is an indirect experience of ourselves mediated by idea rather than by contact, control rather than receptivity. The yamas, though characterized as restraint, actually serve to open us up beyond a restrained existence. Knowing ourselves through self-image only turns us into objects for ourselves. This is unsatisfying. Hidden within the egoic strategies of stealing, being dishonest, or treating others as objects is a much deeper longing obscured by habitual tendency. Our deepest longing, also our greatest fear, is to simply be, without creating a need to be. Every negative behavior is a distorted attempt to connect with something greater than our conditioned circumstances. Thus, waking up in the yoga tradition, especially through the practice of the yamas, is waking up to a life of intimacy.

Any project of the ego is a facsimile of direct experience. The ego is always trying to become something other than it is, and the yamas are the antidote to these ambitions. There is no world beyond our actions here and their eventual effects, no matter how much we try to create something more everlasting, a utopia, a place away from this relational reality. Frustrated by this, we create otherworldly metaphysics, thinking that practice takes us away from this very world when in fact it connects us more deeply to the inherent nonduality of self and world.

> "O Pavamana, place me in that deathless,
> undecaying world wherein the light of heaven
> is set and everlasting luster shines."[1]

These words from the Vedas ring true to the part of us longing (or hoping) for something otherworldly to rescue us from the birth-death-and-birth cycle of existence. We want to create permanence in an impermanent world. The yamas remind us, however, that practice begins in this world, in this body, and nowhere other than right here. You and I are here together, and as such, our relationship forms the basis of the path, not a departure from it. Our relationships are our yoga practice; our practice exists not in some other place at some other time but in this very interconnected existence—you, I, water, trees, cars, winds, and breath. Water lilies and stars, breath and mind, rocks and moss—our stories about reality create separation, when in fact close examination reveals only the interpermeation of forms, coming and going.

The first two limbs, of restraints and ethics, are inseparable from intimacy. What yoga practice entails is not a self-reform or a self-improvement project but a complete forgetting of self-enclosure—an absence of that continuous checking and rechecking of our sense of ourselves. We no longer need check ourselves in the mirror of circumstance, constantly concerned with our place and performance in the scheme of things. We can instead simply be, breathing in and out, taking action based on a direct meeting with and response to our circumstances. But in order to truly meet our circumstances, we need to see them for what they are, and that is why ethics and psychology are bound together as psychological, social, and environmental action.

This eight-limbed path thus sets out to teach us about our patterns of reaction and also suggests appropriate actions, not as commandments but rather as suggestions. After learning about the ways we react, over and over again, we can embark on a project of action. And how do we take action? What do we do? How do we move? What are the conditions for spontaneous action, for feeling whole without needing to *become* "someone"?

There is no final way to act that will be judged as ultimately pure or essentially violent, except by those around us. The yamas are designed to open us up to those around us by motivating us to contemplate our actions of body, speech, and mind, internally and externally. In being sensitive to the effects of our actions, we open to the greater good. The yamas teach us about karma and the consequences of our intentions. When we do not understand the workings of karma, ethical restraints are not treated as psychological tools but rather as commandments or rules.

Again, the ethical practices outlined in this first limb are not to be thought of as commandments that will be punished by an all-powerful god. The nondual traditions, which include yoga, most forms of Buddhism, some schools of Advaita Vedanta, and Taoism, don't operate within a system of rights and wrongs, which, in effect, would turn the theory of karma into a theory of a god who rewards or punishes. Karma is retributive only in its effect on us psychologically, not metaphysically. To add to this, by treating karma as attention to our actions in the here and now, we begin to see that we have the potential for awakening and also the potential for shutting down. Good and bad, heaven and hell, no longer become external or idealistic places or principles but rather psychological potentials. Instead of a divine that determines what is good or bad, we recognize in ourselves the ability to wake up and also the ability to return to a life of habit. When we see these two energies—waking up and closing down—operating in the mind and body at any given moment, we begin to see how important it is that we meditate on our actions of body, speech, and mind.

This continually keeps our practice connected with this world at this moment. "It is important to be responsible for everything you do and to see clearly the effects of your actions," my first yoga teacher said when I asked her the definition of *karma*, "What you do right now counts."

Many yoga students tell me that they cannot take action until they come to a place of stillness in mind. But Patañjali does not teach in this way. Though he may not have known about sticky mats and buckwheat cushions, Patañjali would argue strenuously for the practitioner to see engagement in the world and formal practice on the mat and cushion as one and the same thing. This is where his first limb begins. Abstract ideas about relationship, nonviolence, and ethics are very beautiful and compelling but what use are they in terms of psychological change if they cannot be put into practice?

A center of gravity is finding in oneself and others both the stillness of nonreactivity and the vitality of compassionate and wise action. Yoga is not about passivity; it's about being in the world without being enslaved by worldly identification. The formal practices of these eight limbs help ground the practitioner in a balanced practice that uproots any habits in mind and body that prevent true freedom.

The other limbs, which we will discuss in greater detail later in this book, are also specific forms of practice. *Pratyāhāra* is the practice of naturally internalizing attention; *dhāraṇā* is the mindful practice of returning over and over again to an object of meditation such as the breath, mantra, sound, or sensations in the body; and *dhyāna* is the unfolding of dhāraṇā into a focused and concentrated state of mind. The stillness of dhyāna then becomes the platform from which one practices the several stages of *samādhi*.

Samādhi is not some final resting place, nor is it a goal of yoga, as many assume; rather, samādhi is a technique to be practiced like every other limb in the eight-limbed system. It consists of deepening our meditation practice to the point where we experience firsthand the ultimate separation of pure awareness and that which is impermanent. However, samādhi, as a series of techniques, is also subject to change, and returns us, full cycle, to the practice of ethics described in the first limb. If our ethical commitments as outlined in the yamas are not in good order, our progress in samādhi is stalled, and we backslide to the first limb again. This turns the eight-limbed system into a kind of circular set of practices that eventually form the path of yoga, rather than linear steps that end in samādhi. We continually cycle through the eight limbs, studying and practicing each limb in depth in a kind of circumambulation that wakes us up with each turn.

Cultivating a yoga practice is not just about physical flexibility and strength. Cultivating awareness is not about race, gender, or class—it's about waking up to who we are and our place in the world. That is why we start with the yamas.

The heart of yoga is the cultivation of equilibrium in mind and body so that one can wake up to the reality of being alive, which includes not just joy and health but impermanence, aging, suffering, and death. A yoga practice that excludes the shadows of illness or aging cuts itself off from the truths of being alive. Similarly, a practice that focuses exclusively on physical culture and the performance of yoga poses at the expense of psychological understanding and transformation is a one-sided practice. Without the balanced practice of all eight limbs, and a path rooted in the first limb especially, yoga practice can easily become another form of materialism.

# 8. The Five *Kleṣas*

WHAT PATTABHI JOIS described while touching his heart and speaking of "the enemies of the heart" was a description of the basic symptoms of suffering. "*Saṁsāra hālāhala,*" we often chant before we begin an āsana class. *Hālāhala* refers to the poisonous herb of saṁsāra (conditioned existence) that keeps the wheel of suffering in motion. It's said in this chant that we have swallowed the poisonous herb of habitual existence, and the path of yoga is using the poison as a means of finding our way back to complete sanity. But more important than his description of the symptoms of distress was Pattabhi Jois's later remark about how to work with those symptoms. His reference to the five kleṣas is derived from the *Yoga-Sutra* attributed to Patañjali. After describing duḥkha as a product of repetitive psychological and physical patterns, Patañjali describes the five factors that contribute to putting into motion the wheel of suffering. The five kleṣas are as follows: avidyā (not seeing things as they are), raga (attachment), dveṣa (aversion), asmitā (the story of I, me, and mine), and abhiniveśa (the thirst for further existence).

One of the interesting aspects of considering the six poisons as symptoms of the five kleṣas lies in understanding what we mean by a "symptom." A symptom, by definition, is a characteristic or sign of the existence of something else. The term *symptom* comes from *sym*, "together," and *tom*, "part, piece, or slice." A symptom, like any one of the six poisons—desire, anger, delusion, greed, envy, and sloth—is only a slice of what is actually occurring for someone; on a deeper level we need to look at the root causes of suffering.

The five kleṣas keep suffering in motion because they create loops in the mind-body that reinforce habitual patterns of perception and reaction. They are a concise summation of the basic psychological principles of yoga. The term *kleṣa* comes from the verbal root *klis,* which means "to suffer, torment, or distress."

Let's explore the ways in which these five kleṣas create and reinforce patterns of habit. Perception begins in the sense organs. One cannot perceive the world independent of the sense organs and the mind. All experience is filtered through the sense organs and the mind, and as data comes in through the sense organs, it becomes organized into experience. The term *psychology,* in the context of yoga, can be defined as "the organization of experience," or, more specifically, the way the sense organs and mind organize sense data into subjective experience.

As data moves through the sense organs, we become aware of experience through sensations. We know that there is sensation because there is always a corresponding feeling. Slowing down our experience allows us to notice the ways in which we organize experience. On close inspection, which is what we call "mindfulness," we notice how all sensations give rise to feeling. Feelings can be positive, negative, or neutral. They can be pleasurable or unpleasurable. It's almost as if all sensations in the body fall into one of three buckets: positive, negative, and neutral. For instance, if we are sitting in meditation and feel pain in the knee, we are aware of pain in the knee because we are feeling sensations. In other words, feeling is a mind-body process.

When we feel feelings that are negative, such as pain in the knee, there is usually a corresponding reaction of either attachment (raga) or aversion (dveṣa). Attachment is the desire to repeat pleasurable experience, and aversion is the act of trying to get out of uncomfortable feeling. One can sum up both attachment and aversion under the umbrella term *clinging,* because when you look deeply into attachment, you find aversion to what is not pleasurable. Attachment is aversion to displeasure, and aversion is attachment to pleasure. Aversion is clinging to what is pleasurable. Attachment is the leaning into experience, and aversion is the leaning away from experience. Most of our psychological and physical energy is spent flip-flopping back and forth, moment to moment, between attachment and aversion.

Yoga is the practice of going beyond our habits of creating opposites. When we can remove the deeply ingrained habits of our likes and dislikes by seeing not only how they cause separation but also how we construct and act out these habits, we arrive in a reality prior to separation. Attachment and aversion are always happening to a "me" outside of experience (see diagram 1).

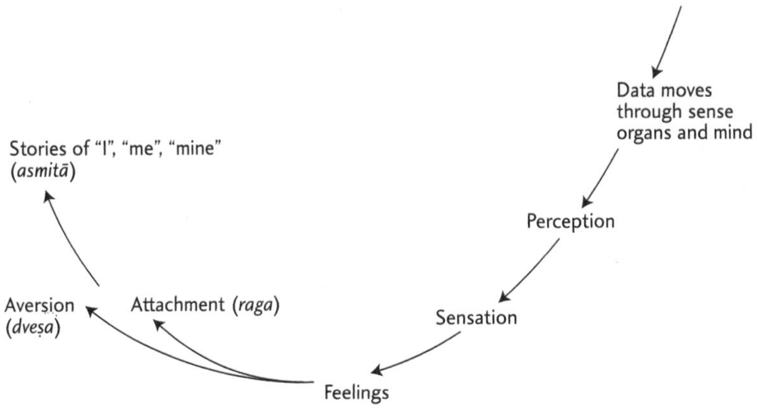


**Diagram 1**

Whenever there is attachment or aversion, there is always the creation of a story of self. This is called "asmitā." For example, if there is pain in the knee, it is experienced as a physical phenomenon, namely a negative feeling, until the moment that there is aversion to the pain. When the aversion to feeling sensation begins, there is a mechanism in the mind that creates a sense of "I" and superimposes this "I" on the unfolding physical experience. There is a movement from feeling pain in the knee to articulating to ourselves pain in the knee as something happening to "me." We say to ourselves, "There is pain in my knee," "I don't like this." In this instinctual moment, an "I" is born that has inserted itself into the phenomenon of pain, but was not initially built into the sensation. In other words, the feeling of pain in "my" knee is an addition to what is unfolding. This is the beginning of duality, because through aversion, a sense of self is created that separates the experience from the one who is experiencing.

Asmitā, the experience of an "I, me, and mine" comes from a mechanism in the mind called the *ahaṇkāra.* This word comes from the verbal root *kṛ,* meaning "action" or "to make," and *aham,* which means "I." It is best translated as the "'I'-maker," and can be thought of as a mechanism in the mind that creates a story of self that is constructed on top of any phenomenon of feeling occurring moment to moment.

Asmitā, the "I"-maker, as a mechanism that gives rise to the feeling of "I, me, and mine" can, for practical purposes, be conceived of as a storyteller. When you contemplate your own thinking process, you may come to notice that almost all of your thoughts are stories about you! Most of us go through the day telling ourselves endless stories about ourselves. Our perception in daily life seems to pivot around this ongoing narrative of "me." We talk to others about ourselves, and if there is no one around, we talk to ourselves about ourselves and call it thinking!

Many scholars translate *ahaṇkāra* as "the ego." However, Freud's definition of the ego is that which mediates between conscious and unconscious, internal and external, personal and social, and is considered, in his theory, to be the center of the personality. In yoga psychology, the "I"-maker is a cause of suffering (kleṣa), because it is constantly filtering our experience in a self-centered way. This takes Freud's idea of narcissism much farther. It's not so much that we have fallen for our image of ourselves; rather we are constantly overlaying each moment with a story of self, preventing a direct experience of reality, creating a case of mistaken identity! Furthermore, compassion, listening, or the ability to take in others is always superseded by the aggressive mechanism of the "I"-maker.

Down the road from my house at a local photocopy shop there is on a table with staplers and pens an enormous elastic-band ball—green and blue and red and very dense. When you take one band, wrap it around another, over which you wrap another band, and so on, after a while the ball grows larger and tighter. The personality is like an elastic-band ball: the wider the diameter, the more dense the core. Our stories of ourselves wrap one over another, creating conceptions of self that we fail to see as conceptions. Instead, we think of ourselves not as stories wrapped around other stories, but as fixed and somewhat permanent entities. As we age, the stories we tell about ourselves, much like the elastics on the circumference of a ball, have to be stretched wider and longer in order to wrap around our previous conceptions of self. If we imagine the self as an elastic-band ball that is getting larger, we can see how the more we create stories of self, the more the core of the self feels real. The center of an elastic-band ball is under great pressure. It is tightly wound and feels more like structure than elastic process. The stories of the self give us the impression that the self actually exists, but at bottom, it's simply an unstable cognition. The imagination uses the raw material of life to create narrative structures that serve to further entrench our belief in a solid and stable entity called "me."

The next kleṣa is abhiniveśa, which is most often understood as the fear of death. However, when you contemplate death, and the corresponding fear that arises whenever you think about death, you begin to see that what you fear most is not that your body is going to decompose or that your hair is going to burn up in flames, it's that "I" am going to die. This story of "me," this anthology of "I," comes to an end. Whether you believe in a future life or not, these chapters of "I" that you've been writing from moment to moment and that you're most thoroughly invested in will come to an end. Since you can't know for certain what happens at the threshold of death (or even in the next moment, for that matter), the mechanism of the "I"-maker begins to speculate, out of existential fear, since it knows not what will occur beyond that door. Even when you feel lonely and alone, who is actually alone?

Abhiniveśa is not the fear of the death of the body per se, but the fear of letting go of the story of "me." The purpose of meditation is to watch the process of clinging and thus gain insight into impermanence, which has, as an effect, psychological stillness. The very same phenomena that dominate our lives and actions when we're unaware of them are seen to be impermanent and insubstantial in the light of awareness. Abhiniveśa cuts to the heart of our attempts at permanence. At the moment of death, we can no longer hold on to our conceptions of self. Palliative-care workers describe, time and time again, the difficult process of dying for someone who clings incessantly to their ideas of themselves, others, or life in general.

Why wait until the moment of death to let go of these constructions of self when we can do so in every moment? Paradoxically, we hold on because we see that these stories of "I, me, and mine" keep us at a safe and conceptual distance from reality, which gives us the illusion of comfort, existential security, and permanence. This illusion is called avidyā. The Sanskrit *vidyā,* as described before, becomes the Latin word *vidéo,* which in English becomes the word *video,* meaning "to see." The prefix *a* turns any word in Sanskrit into its opposite. *Avidyā,* therefore, refers to the inability to see things or be with things as they are. *Avidyā* describes not being engaged with life as it unfolds and passes away. Why can't we be present with life? We can't see things as they are (vidyā) because of our habitual patterns of attachment and aversion. This is an amazing and troubling aspect of our human condition. We already exist as people in the here and now, yet we still try to construct ourselves as "selves" in the present moment, and find ourselves missing the present moment completely.

There is a joke in yoga that asks, "If you had to hide something that was the most valuable thing you had, where would you hide it?" The answer is: "in the present moment." If you hide something in the present moment, no one will be able to find it. Most of the time we are not present or engaged with things as they are (vidyā), because we are so caught in deep grooves of raga (attachment), dveṣa (aversion), and our stories of self (asmitā).

Since we take actions (karma) based on these habituated patterns of attachment and aversion, we reinforce in the mind and body those same patterns. The effects of our actions leave residues in the mind-body. These residues are called *saṁskāras*. Saṁskāras are the psychological and physical grooves that influence the way we perceive each moment of experience based on previous actions. The saṁskāras groove and condition our organs of perception. Therefore, the actions that we take, and their particular consequences, create in the mind and body predispositions to perceive and act in each moment in habitual and conditioned ways (as illustrated in diagram 2). This completes the cycle of saṁsāra, illustrating the turning wheel of suffering.

What is important to remember is that while this cycle is descriptive of a state of dissatisfaction, it is a cycle open to change. The underlying structure of the brain and the basic substratum of the body itself are both changing all the time. Always in motion, the brain and body are structurally unstable, which accounts for the flexibility and elasticity of our human organism. Not only do our conditions change, our conditioning can change as well.

To illustrate the way the basic patterns of mind and body (saṁskāras) change, imagine the film of a camera. Imagine that the film represents your mind, brain, and body. Now imagine using the camera to take a picture of a tree. When a picture is taken, the film is exposed to new information—that of the image of a tree. In order for the image to be retained, the film must react to the light and "change" to record the image of the tree. Similarly, in order for new patterns of behavior and

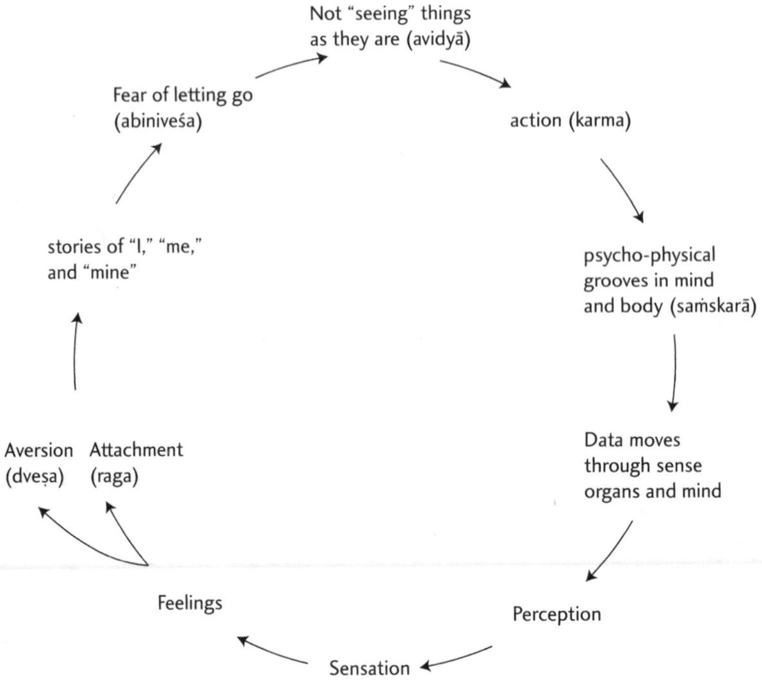


**Diagram 2**

action to be retained in memory, changes in the mind-body representing the new knowledge must occur.

Looking back at diagram 2, we see that not only is this a description of suffering, it is also descriptive of the psychology of addiction, because the mind-body circulates the same patterns through repetition, reinforcing repetitive choices and actions. While presenting this model to a group of psychiatrists at a conference on mind and body, one doctor described this as "cognitive behavioral therapy on steroids!" This model describes not only our addiction to that which on the surface causes us distress or discontent—such as habits of smoking, drugs, gambling, or sex—but, on a more subtle and profound level, articulates our addiction to creating stories of self. At the core of any addiction lies the addiction to a story.

Yoga psychology pushes us to see through the addictive tendency to create stories of ourselves by representing ourselves to ourselves in order to make us feel real. But this reality is an illusion. The self is nothing more than a conglomeration of stories stretched out and overlapping one another like the giant elastic-band ball. Let's use an example.

Suppose we are at home alone and after finishing household chores, making a meal, checking e-mail, and engaging in other distractions, we begin to feel lonely. Perhaps this loneliness is accompanied by a feeling of boredom and then sadness. This is not an uncommon experience. As the feelings of loneliness and sadness fill our awareness, the tendency in the mind is to look for a way out of these negative feelings. Instead of allowing these feelings to arise, we turn to the freezer, take out a pint of ice cream, and finish the pint faster than we realize. (You can substitute in this example whatever your common avoidance strategy is.)

After finishing the ice cream in a state of numbness and dissociation, we begin to feel a threefold feeling. Firstly, we feel physically terrible for having eating an entire pint of ice cream. Second, there is usually a degree of shame or self-judgment for having indulged in this reactive pattern. Third, the feelings of sadness and loneliness that we tried to avoid with the ice cream return again. Freud called this "the return of the repressed." And as Einstein said, energy is neither created nor destroyed, it just changes form. In other words, our attempts to escape the feelings that we have determined unacceptable only fuels further feelings that in turn reinforce our habits even further. What we push away always returns with the same amount of force we expended to keep it at bay.

What would happen if instead of going to the freezer when experiencing the growing or even acute feelings of sadness or loneliness, we sat down and paid attention to our breath? Yoga asks us to stay with feelings without seeking to avoid them. This does not mean dwelling in or indulging feelings indefinitely—such an approach can turn into another form of storytelling. Rather, it means that we stay patiently and with an attitude of acceptance with whatever is occurring in the present moment as it arises, unfolds, and passes away. Just put your body there.

Instead of going to the freezer, allow whatever feelings are arising to unfold, however uncomfortable, in order for them to be felt fully and eventually let go of.

Staying present with feelings—especially negative feelings, such as physical or emotional pain—requires an attitude of patience and intentional acceptance. Breathing with uncomfortable feelings requires both steadiness and ease and the ability to explore our experience without judgment or distraction. Mindful awareness is nonconceptual, nonjudgmental, sometimes nonverbal, and exploratory. Pure awareness is not the extinguishing of the self but rather the stilling of the construction of the story of "me" as it arises. The stilling of these fluctuating stories is not the goal of yoga but rather the final technique by means of which we can wake up to the reality of a present moment not obscured by self. This is where the path of yoga begins. The mystic Kabir describes the way in which habitual conditioning and our preoccupation with ourselves has the tendency to hijack our spiritual practice:

> Friend, please tell me what I can do about this world
> I hold on to, and keep spinning out!
>
> I gave up sewn clothes, and wore a robe,
> But I noticed one day the cloth was well woven.
>
> So I bought some burlap, but I still
> Throw it elegantly over my left shoulder.
>
> I pulled back my sexual longings,
> And now I discover that I'm angry a lot.
>
> I gave up rage, and now I notice
> That I'm greedy all day.
>
> I worked hard at dissolving the greed,
> And now I'm proud of myself.

While the mind wants to break its link with the world,
It still holds on to one thing![1]

Like a magnetic force, the habit of orienting our experience around the axiom of "I, me, and mine" is extremely difficult to undo, because as an addictive habit, it has great momentum. So the first step is to witness how the mechanism operates from moment to moment, and there are practical ways of doing this.

The first step of extinguishing this cycle of satisfaction-dissatisfaction is to use the power of naming, which is a linguistic tool of the mind. The mechanism of using language to name (*nama*) something is called *buddhi*. The term *buddhi* means "intelligence" and is where the mind can recognize something through language. Language allows us to recognize our experience, and usually when we are caught up in something, it is hard to name it. Therefore, naming acts as a way of finding the right distance from sensory objects (*ālambana*) as they appear in awareness so that we can notice what is there rather than slipping into reactivity. There is a difference between naming something and telling stories about it. Language helps us orient ourselves to the object of awareness, and once there, we drop into feeling without storytelling. When we give up our stories, we can usually feel experience with much greater sensitivity, compassion, and clarity. Nonattachment does not mean dissociation; it actually connotes connection and engagement with what is. Nonattachment does not prevent compassion; it sets up the conditions for it.

When we are in a difficult yoga pose, as an example, and pain arises in the legs, we stay with the pain by reminding ourselves to stay with leg, hip, breath, and so on, rather than telling ourselves the same habitual stories we usually tell when faced with strong sensations. So naming is a powerful tool that helps us recognize and investigate our experience. But once it has been named, we don't proliferate the moment with stories; rather we remain present with whatever is (see diagram 3).

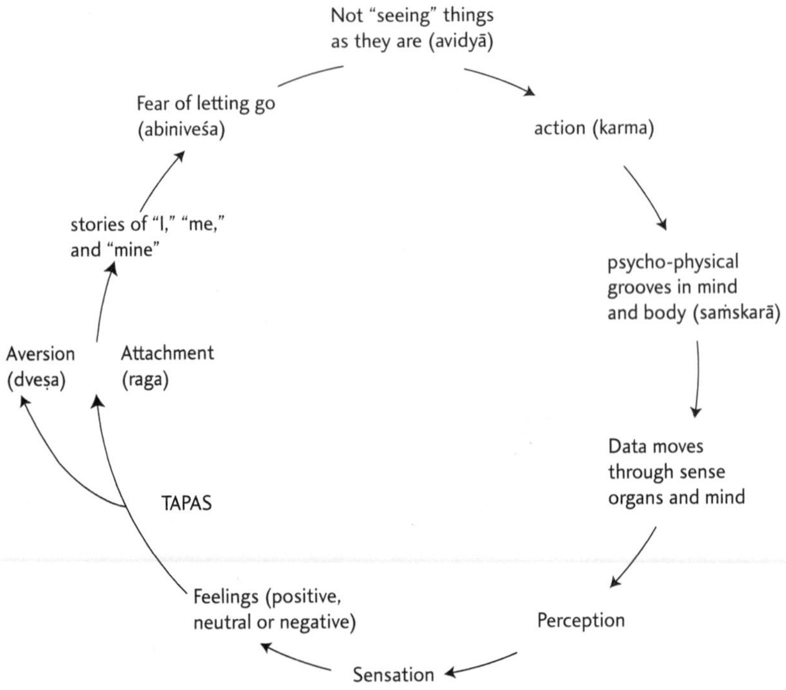


**Diagram 3**

## Tapas

When we stay with feelings in mind-body, whether emotional or physical or both, we are in a way staying in the tension of opposites. This is called "tapas." When we can stay with a feeling without attachment or aversion, we experience the practice of tapas. Traditionally, the term *tapas* referred in Vedic times to the fire at the center of a sacrificial ritual. In the Vedas, rituals revolved around sacrifices, in which, through the burning of various objects, a symbolic offering to the gods secured one a beneficial place in future existence. Over time, the term *tapas* took on a more subtle meaning. In the Upaniṣads, *tapas* refers to austerity, concentrated discipline, penance, or heat. The term was used to refer to a student who is burning with aspiration or a practitioner who is burning with intensity to know the truth. In the *Yoga-Sutra,* however, it took on a more psychological meaning: the heat of staying in the tension of opposites.

In any given moment, we can meet that moment with the conditioned habits of attachment and aversion, or we can meet that moment with spontaneity and freedom from conditioned responses. Carl Jung defined *tapas* as the "transcendent function," which refers to the creative moment that occurs when we stay in the tension of opposites. *Tapas,* therefore, can be defined as "patience." The practice of tapas is a practice of patience.

When we perpetuate the realm of binary thinking—likes and dislikes, me and mine, inner and outer—we fail to embody the root meaning of yoga—the ultimate interconnection and nonseparation of existence. This is not a reality without feeling or a life dissociated from the world but rather the ability to be fully engaged in life with the ability to experience fully its impact. Tapas is being grounded in a reality that is not "apart from," and the skill of "grounding" is the activity of feeling *what is* without plotting escape routes. It is the ability to stand still in difficulty that makes new ground. Patience and stillness strengthen the very ground we stand on.

The work of tapas, which is the essence of yoga, is the cultivation of the skills that allow us to be present in the here and now with whatever is occurring, whether positive, negative, or neutral. Yoga is the instrument by which we hold ourselves in the fire of habit until we burn away that which averts the heat of change. Staying with habit and the paradoxical discomfort of letting go is what not only contains the process of yoga but fuels it. Pantañjali says it's a great victory when you can experience a feeling as a feeling. In other words, eventually through this practice we can begin to experience feelings as feelings—impersonal phenomena as opposed to feelings in the form of explosive dramas of "I, me, and mine." Feeling is the key to the present moment. It anchors us in experience.

Staying present in any moment of experience creates new patterns in the mind-body. To illustrate this in terms of psychophysiology, imagine making an impression of a coin in a lump of clay. In order for the impression of the coin to appear in the clay, changes must occur in the clay—the shape of the clay changes as the coin is pressed into it. Similarly, the neural circuitry of the brain, the pathways of the breath and nervous system, and the anatomy of the body must organize in response to new experience or sensory stimulation. Whenever there is a moment of nonreactivity, this is a moment of action. This is the action of nonaction. Whatever you reflect on frequently becomes, over time, the basic inclination of your mind. Not reacting in habitual ways creates new patterns, which in effect create new and more wholesome patterns of mind, body, and speech. This is the physiology of karma. Every action has an effect, even the action of nondoing.

Tapas is the key to yoga because being able to sit in the midst of opposition creates the heat necessary for change; yoga occurs when we let opposites move right through our pores, only to see that opposition is a conceptual designation that falls away when we are with the energy of the moment rather than with our storytelling. In patient openness, what was habit and immobility becomes receptivity and the capacity to open to experience. Whether this paradox is in the alignment of yoga postures, internal and external rotation in the leg bones, feeling the space between the in-breath and the out-breath, or the cultivation of stillness when habit pulls us into its familiar arms, it is paradox that creates new opportunity. Yoga occurs in paradox when, through tapas, two opposing energies have lost their pull and reveal a completeness. When our attention is on the relationship between opposing energies, they lose their oppositional tension, because we focus on their relations, not their substantiality.

## *Freedom from Duḥkha*

Reviewing the diagram that depicts the wheel of suffering, Patañjali asks the practitioner to consider what can be removed from this cycle and still have a functioning, healthy human engaged in relationship? The answer for Patañjali (as illustrated in diagram 4) is to slice the wheel in half.

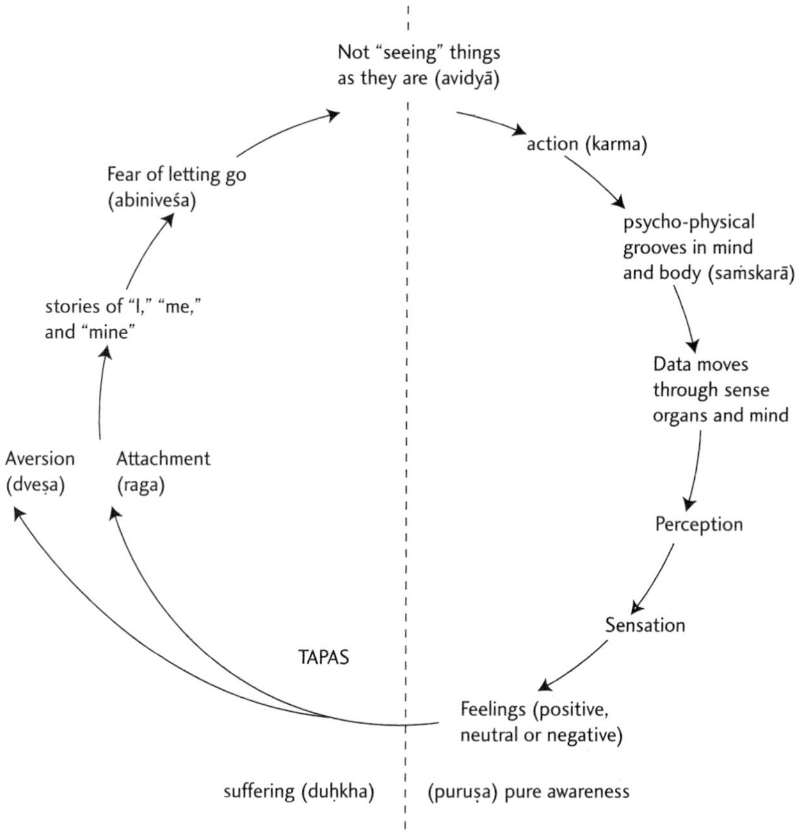


**Diagram 4**

Instead of reacting to feelings, we pay attention to what is occurring in the present moment and, in doing so, take actions that reinforce patterns in the mind-body that create the conditions for being just as present in the next moment. In contemporary neuroscience, this is called "neuroplasticity." Neuroplasticity sees the brain as an organ not separated from mind or body, and describes the brain's ability to reorganize itself by forming new neural connections throughout life. By sprouting new nerve endings, the brain constantly changes within the context of its environment. It is not a closed system. Like the theory of the saṁksāras, the mind-body is not a closed loop. Our habits, predispositions, attitudes, and behaviors are open and flexible systems constantly in motion, subject to change, and they grow increasingly complex in order to become more and more efficient.

We expend so much energy running away from reality. Most of us are familiar with mind states that operate like closed circuits, perhaps repetitive cycles of addiction or ways of arguing with loved ones that seem infinite in their repetitive cycles. We know, too, what it is like to be lost in thoughts of past or future over and over again. The key in the model of the five kleṣas is that though the mind-body is contracted in states of addiction and delusion, this self-centered and inflexible posture is not permanent. A moment of suffering can also become a path out of suffering. The very intensity of each one of the kleṣas, when experienced fully, pushes us into seeing where the mind is fixed and to what it is holding on. Unlike the detached state of pulling away from experience, nonattachment creates flexibility by bringing us closer to what is actually occurring, even as we are less encumbered by our viewpoint. Relaxing the heart when we see contracted states arising disentangles us from the web of self-identification.

Yoga practice is about expanding and strengthening circuits in the mind-body that are less frequently used, and repatterning those that are inefficient. This is called "nirodha." Nirodha is the releasing of habitual patterns or fluctuations in mind-body, but it also describes the energy that comes from that letting go of old patterns.

In yoga, instead of taking a pilgrimage to a particular mountain or temple, we take pilgrimage inside of our own bodies. For most people, this is a more difficult pilgrimage. To walk through the landscape of the body open to feeling whatever feelings arise puts us in touch with the core of the body. However, there are many psychological, emotional, and physical holding patterns in the center of the body that make this pilgrimage difficult. That difficulty is also our potential for liberation.

If we look at diagram 5, on the left-hand side we see a model of duḥkha (from attachment/aversion all the way to avidyā), and on the right-hand side we see a model of a personality free from the constraints of a condi-

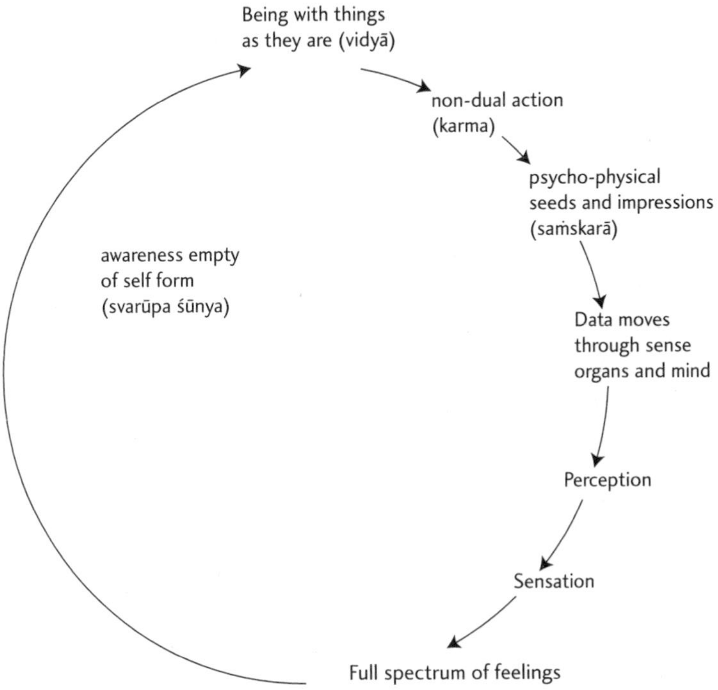


**Diagram 5**

tioned existence of stress and discontent. On the left-hand side, we see a constructed and illusory clinging to self; on the right-hand side we see the spontaneous expression of a personality free from the need to create self. When you no longer need to create a sense of self, you are free to

# 9. Freedom through the *Kleṣas*

> Wherever your mind applies its full power of attention, there you make a seat for yourself.
>
> —*Rig-Veda*

THE FIVE KLEṢAS teach us that by putting a wedge between our feelings and our aversion or attachment to them, we make a seat for ourselves in present experience. Letting go of a self-centered response to reality brings us into a more realistic, clear, and grounded relationship with life, which manifests in intelligent action. At first this may seem like a paradox or a game of games. In a certain way, it is. By saying that there is a falling away of the construction of self, we are not saying that there is no self. We are simply saying that "self" construction is seen through. We are not trying to eliminate narrative. Human beings love to tell stories. What this model proposes is that what creates suffering is not seeing our stories of ourselves as stories. Patañjali describes two methods for moving from a cycle of duḥkha to a cycle of freedom. The first is *abhyāsa,* which is the cultivation of new patterns in the mind and body, and second is *vairāgya,* which is the letting go of habitual patterns. For example, one of the dominant stories of self in contemporary Western culture is self-judgment. According to this model, our work as practitioners is to monitor the quality of our awareness, which means catching the stories of self-judgment as they unfold. When we catch ourselves in a story of self-judgment, we practice abhyāsa, which in essence means cultivating a kinder and more compassionate story to break down the tendency toward self-judgment. Abhyāsa refers to letting go of the story of self-judgment by seeing through it. Again, we see a story as a story, and in seeing a pattern as a pattern, we create just enough distance from the pattern that we can see it for what it is and let it go.

Many people respond to this dropping of the story of self by saying that this can occur only for those who have a strong sense of self and that people with low self-esteem *need* to construct a story of self. Many modern therapeutic formulas to work with low self-esteem have failed because they are simply replacing one story of self with another. The problem that begins in the mechanism of the "I"-maker is primarily the clinging to a singular narrative. It turns out that people with low self-esteem are very attached to their story of self. In fact, many people with low self-esteem cling more to their identification to their stories of self than people who are inflated. Low self-esteem is the identification with a very specific narrative of self. All clinging to notions of self reify that which is ultimately unknowable and empty. Heinz Kohut, one of the great psychoanalytic theorists of the last century, in his groundbreaking work, *The Restoration of the Self,* writes,

> My investigation contains hundreds of pages dealing with the psychology of the self—yet it never assigns an inflexible meaning to the term self, it never explains how the essence of the self should be defined. But I admit this fact without contrition or shame. The self . . . is, like all reality . . . not knowable in its essence. We cannot, by introspection and empathy, penetrate the self per se; only its introspectively or empathically perceived psychological manifestations are open to us.[1]

While there is a sense of self in psychological or "introspective" terms, the actuality of an abiding essence that is traceable back to some particular source, entity, or substance is nowhere to be found. The self is a *story* of self.

## *Dropping the Narrative*

Yoga psychology is a series of techniques that interrupt all forms of attachment, especially our attachment to self. In the second limb articulated by Patañjali in the second chapter of the *Yoga-Sutra,* he describes *svādhyāya* (self-study) as a method of seeing through our attachments. It's important to remember that self-study does not refer only to self-reflection but to the investigation of the nature of constructing a self to begin with. We are not as interested in the manifestation of self as we are in the need to construct a self at all. This is the work of dropping the story line. When we contemplate that which we cling to most, we find, embedded in the deepest and most condensed recesses of the personality, elaborate narratives. Narrative implicitly assumes causality, that such and such happened causing a certain result. But the logic of narrative—and Indian myths point this out over and over again—is always flawed by the basic fact that a narrative is simply a narrative. A story is just a story, and though we may call our stories scientific theory, theology, psychology, or even self, they are still constructed attempts at linguistic description and expression. The construction is what is important. This is well illustrated in a famous story about Kṛṣṇa:

Kṛṣṇa comes to earth in the form of a young boy. Like many young boys, he is playing with other kids and eating dirt. Out of the corner of her eye, his mother catches him eating dirt, and asks, "Kṛṣṇa, are you eating dirt again?" To which he responds, with his mouth closed, "Mmm-mmmmm, no."

Again she asks, "Kṛṣṇa, are you eating dirt?"

And with a mouthful of dirt he turns away. One of the other children with whom Kṛṣṇa is playing turns to Kṛṣṇa's mother and says, "Yes, Kṛṣṇa is eating dirt."

Immediately, as any mother would do, Kṛṣṇa's mother pulls him out of the group and away from the rest of the kids, then forcefully opens his mouth to find his gums, teeth, and tongue embedded with dirt. With her hands holding his mouth open, she peers in a little farther, and behind the root of his palate, she sees a familiar darkness. As if looking into a blackened night sky she focuses again. Then, within that darkness, she sees the bright moon, a sky of stars, moving constellations, and then sees herself as Kṛṣṇa's mother, and passes out. Amid the dust and profundity of her vision, she lies on the ground unconscious.

Seeing his mother passed out, Kṛṣṇa kneels down in the sand, and waves over her the illusion that she is his mother. She then wakes up, feeling herself again as Kṛṣṇa's mother, and everything is OK; she returns again to the responsibility and safety of her role and her place in the fabric of her culture.

In calling her son away from kids who are eating dirt, Kṛṣṇa's mother exemplifies the typical and relative relationship of mother and son. There is no denying in this circumstance that Kṛṣṇa's mother is acting out the instinctual role of motherhood and that Kṛṣṇa, in eating dirt, is being a young boy. This is the relative world of mother and son. When Kṛṣṇa's mother looks into her son's mouth and sees the stars and the moon, this represents the mystical experience that is, in essence, direct experience of the present moment. It represents the falling away of all of Kṛṣṇa's mother's attachments, perspectives, and views, only to reveal her most cherished attachment: identification with the role of mother. For most parents, this is one of our most cherished attachments—being a parent. However, Kṛṣṇa does not belong to his mother. On a relative level, Kṛṣṇa is her son. But on an ultimate level, Kṛṣṇa's mother gains insight into the truth that nothing belongs to "I, me, or mine." However, this is too much for her to bear, so she passes out.[2]

In other versions of this story, Kṛṣṇa tries these games over and over, yet in all these stories, Kṛṣṇa's mother never lets go of her attachment to herself as a mother. This paradox demonstrates the complexity of nonattachment in the realm of human relationship. Our mind creates stories of self and other, strung up on banners in consciousness, and although those advertisements feel real, they are actually patterns of skywriting that dissolve into nothing.

Even our parents, children, lovers, or friends are not and can never be "I, me, or mine." Even at a physiological level, Kṛṣṇa is *of* the mother but does not *belong* to the mother. On a biological level, the story of Kṛṣṇa eating dirt touches the heart of our relational existence. This is described clearly by the physician Hélène Rouche in an interview with the philosopher Luce Irigaray:

> First, I'll remind you of what the placenta is: It's a tissue, formed by the embryo, which, while being closely imbricated with the uterine mucosa remains separate from it. This has to be reiterated, because there's a commonly held belief view that the placenta is a mixed formation, half-maternal, half-fetal. However, although the placenta is a formation of the embryo, it behaves like an organ that is practically independent of it. It plays a mediating role on two levels. On the one hand, it's the mediating space between mother and fetus, which means that there's never a fusion of maternal and embryonic tissues. On the other hand, it constitutes a system regulating exchanges between the two organisms, not merely quantitatively regulating the exchanges (nutritious substances from mother to fetus, waste matter in the other direction), but also modifying the maternal metabolism. . . . It thus establishes a relationship between mother and fetus, enabling the latter to grow without exhausting the mother in the process, and yet not simply being a means for obtaining nutrition.[3]

The placenta, continues Hélène, also takes over from the ovary itself by producing steroids that go to both mother and infant. How this relates to the leash of asmitā is profound: The division of a "you" and "me" and the belief that we can appropriate an other or even belong completely to an other is physiologically inaccurate. The relative autonomy of the placenta ensures the growth in one body of another body.[4] Biological and psychological reality intertwine here. One could almost say that the placenta acts as an agent that maintains not only the separation of the infant and mother but their mutual interdependence as well. It's not that Kṛṣṇa is not the son of his mother, it's that the relationship and the nonbelonging go together. The role of the placenta makes the actuality of a child in a womb seem more like a transplant than anything willed by the parent or infant.[5]

This is more than just a simple paradox, it is a negotiation between what is mine and what is other. The kleṣas implore us to see that there is no solid "I" to be found anywhere that is eternal. The "self" that we want to hang on to as something fixed and everlasting is a misplaced desire, one that maintains the momentum of satisfaction-dissatisfaction because nothing conceptualized as eternal provides ultimate security, even if that conceptualization feels real. The placenta example does not describe a state of fusion but an organized economy of relationship. Yet to say there is no self is also to fall to one side of the spectrum, and is therefore also incorrect. At the moment of birth, once the child exits the mother's body, the placenta departs as well, not belonging either to mother or infant yet supportive of and contingent on the survival of both.

Returning to diagrams 4 and 5 of the five kleṣas from the last chapter, we can see that any form of attachment or aversion not only constructs a clinging narrative of self, it also never fails to create the conditions for dissatisfaction. The storyteller is always searching for a way to superimpose itself on experience. Why? Because whenever there is storytelling, whenever there is a construction of self, there is always anxiety. This anxiety is existential in nature. It is existential because the storyteller knows at some basic level that without its ongoing functioning things go along much smoother. When Pattabhi touched his heart while taking a deep breath, he was pointing to the kleṣas as the five enemies that keep the heart from opening. An open heart, a human simply being, immediately presents a manifestation in nature of just being; to simply be without the separation caused by the five kleṣas allows the heart to remain open to the inherent change and flux of life, without clinging and its consequent stress. To feel without getting out of the feeling, no matter how joyful or painful, is to be in touch with the pulse of life. Even a broken heart is an open heart.

The practicality of this for the yoga practitioner is obvious. Vidyā means being with what is. Vidyā means noticing how a thing changes as we observe patiently. Does it continue, is it permanent, to whom or what does it belong? If the self is fictional and not a static and eternal entity, we can begin to embrace it as such. The poet Wallace Stevens describes this kind of psychological freedom in his work "Adagia": "The final belief is to believe in a fiction, which you know to be a fiction, there being nothing else. The exquisite truth is to know that it is a fiction and that you believe in it willingly."[6]

Our work as yoga practitioners is to breathe our circumstances. Avidyā is the mistaken conception that anything can provide permanent satisfaction or ongoing security. Mistaken conception leads to mistaken perception. If we are confined to a representational reality, we are always bound to our theories of reality rather than direct perception through the senses and mind.

# 10. Stillness and Movement

IN MOST YOGA CLASSES, we practice the physical practice of postures and breathing, and the psychological aspects of yoga are not mentioned. The mind, even though its habits are everywhere in physical movement, is an allusive absence, and psychology is rendered "philosophy" and left out of class. Perhaps this has always been the case. It's easy to idealize the cultures of India and Tibet and assume that all yoga practitioners were doing subtle psychological work. It's hard for us to say that "every" practitioner "got it"! What is hidden in history is conjectural from our present day, and it's difficult to be psychic historians and see from the inside how yoga was being practiced and taught. However, we know that from these cultures, highly evolved texts, practices, and teachings arose from practitioners who were able to, as Erich Schiffmann says, "move into stillness."[1] Breath, mind, stillness, and movement were always intertwined in order to study the mind-body and the way out of discontent.

What we mean by "stillness" is psychological stillness. We tend to the body and its infinite layers and our spreading of breath throughout these layers without being apart from the experience. We use the experience to wake up. We use the body to study the mind and the mind to study the body so that we come to see the inherent interpermeation of mind and body and world.

Pushing practice a step farther, we come to see that the body is always changing, energy always blooming, and mind always thinking.

Thoughts are endless. But underneath all that movement there is complete stillness; our conditioning is more flexible, our minds more elastic, our habits more pliable than we ever thought. But going deeper into the psychology of yoga requires the cultivation of an attention span that can rest in stillness rather than moving through the ongoing distortions of habit.

If there is an historical pattern in the evolution of yoga, as judged by texts such as the *Yoga-Sutra* or the *Hatha Yoga Pradīpika,* or even the miraculous *Bhagavad Gītā,* it's that when yoga becomes overly physical, lost in ritual and mere physical achievement, there is always a backlash, a return to the deeper mental elements that complement a meditation on the body. When we look deeply into the body, we find the mind. When we look into the nature of mind, we find nothing other than the "stuff" of life—changing, interconnected, vibrating, and without absolute structure.

The yoga community evolving in the West, especially the network of studios offering public classes, is in a phase of struggle. Students want to deepen their practice, and are usually only offered physical study or esoteric philosophy. Of course this is a grand generalization, but we find little in classes and workshops in the way of psychology. However, it is precisely our ability to work with the mind that contemporary practitioners need most, because it is in the mind that we find our deepest troubles and anxieties. Texts such as the *Yoga-Sutra* are psychology textbooks, pointing the way toward liberation from duḥkha. You do not have to choose physical or psychological practice—they are two parts of a greater whole. As practice matures, it expands horizontally, across all eight limbs, so that you begin to explore the role of the mind in any meditation on physical reality, and conversely, you begin to meditate on the empty nature of physical reality when studying the mind.

When you are able to still some of the patterns of reaction and distraction, duality dissolves, because behind a "me" and "my experience" is what is. You may have your own particular tendencies, but your thoughts are all put together by thoughts. Pure awareness is not personal. Not much is. Even your body is the result of a greater past. One cannot penetrate the "yoga" of yoga—the inherent oneness of reality—if you are preoccupied with yourself. If there is any prejudice, self-judgment, or preconceived idea about you or life in general, the practice is still moving in habit. So we need to get to know that habit, but habit does not dissolve easily. As we move with habit, seeing it for what it is, we can put aside our preferences and take in something greater than our "selves." This is the root of saṁsāra and the route beyond saṁsāra. Beneath all of our ideas and expectations is a constant flow of homeless feelings and thoughts, images and sensations, flowing endlessly and without a structure that holds it together in an everlasting way. It's only when we pick up those ongoing patterns as "I, me, and mine" that such structure is born, and so too is duḥkha.

Yoga becomes more subtle as we continually observe and feel with great attention, with patience and without comment, without assuming any strong attitude toward the object of our observation. If we are meditating on bodiness or mind "stuff," we feel and watch, witness and learn, with openness to what is arising and passing away in the present moment. When we accept what is in this very moment, without pushing or pulling, when there is no running after or running away, we find in our practice a level of deep acceptance and peace. In this way there is no mind observing a body. There is simply the unfolding nature of nature, coming and going. Every posture instruction becomes another route for awareness, another stretch of intelligence. With an attitude of kindness and nonviolence, yoga practice matures internally. Whatever we feel we feel. Whatever we think we think. When we create space enough for feelings and thoughts to come and go in this container of mind and body, meditation occurs spontaneously. Sankaraçarya declares: "One should know that a real posture is that in which the meditation of reality [Brahman] flows spontaneously and unceasingly, and not any other . . ."[2]

# 11. The Five *Kośas*:

## SHEATHS OF THE MIND AND BODY

YOGA IS ESSENTIALLY CONCERNED with teaching us to perceive and respond to reality in such a way that we can transform our perceptions and responses so that the experience of suffering is resolved. While this process may lead to asking legitimate philosophical, psychological, and religious questions, such questions are of secondary concern. The aim of the yoga path is to recognize suffering in its various manifestations and conditions and to cultivate the skills necessary to bring suffering to an end. As Pattabhi Jois emphatically explained in his description of the enemies in the heart, there are five factors that contribute to the experience of suffering and stress, namely, not being with things as they are (avidyā), attachment (raga), aversion (dveṣa), the stories of "I, me, and mine" (asmitā), and the fear of letting go (abhiniveśa).

One of the best ways of seeing how the contributing causes of suffering operate is through a contemplation of the mind-body, and one of the best ways of approaching the mind-body is through the lens of the five kośas. The five kośas are a kind of magnifying glass or prism through which we can better understand the workings and interaction of perception, consciousness, feeling, breathing, and physiology. In addition, the kośas become a meditative tool through which we can undo the habits of the five kleṣas. On the surface, the kośas describe the layers of mind and body and how they interact. On a deeper level, when one practices the last four limbs of meditation, the kośas become a set of strategies for how one should focus one's attention and where, a kind of sequential logic for meditative practice.

Some Hatha Yoga teachers, such as B.K.S. Iyengar, use the kośas as a way of demonstrating how the various layers of mind and body not only interpenetrate but also operate consciously or unconsciously depending on where our awareness is. Iyengar uses detailed mechanical and metaphorical instructions as meditation techniques that assist the practitioner in sensing the various factors that comprise mind and body. This helps get the mind focused on the gross and subtle aspects of a yoga posture and all of the layers in between. Describing what constitutes the mind and body, B.K.S. Iyengar writes that mind and body as a whole "consist of five inter-penetrating and inter-dependent sheaths."[1]

The *Paingala Upaniṣad* describes the koṣas clearly:

> The five sheaths are made of vital air, mind, understanding and bliss. What is brought into being only by the essence of food, what grows only by food, that which finds rest in earth full of the essence of food, that is the sheath made of food, annamaya kośa. That alone is the gross body. The five vital airs, along with the organs of action, constitute the sheath made of the vital principle, prāṇamaya kośa. Mind, along with the organs of perception, is the sheath made of mind, manomaya kośa. The understanding, along with the organs of perception, is the sheath made of intelligence, vijñanamaya kośa. These three sheaths (of life, mind, and intelligence) form the subtle body. The knowledge of one's own form is of the sheath made of bliss, ānandamaya kośa. That is also the causal body.

There are several different sheaths that constitute what we call the mind-body. When we practice yoga postures, meditation, and prāṇāyāma, we are consciously or unconsciously working with these various sheaths, depending on the quality and place of attention. Our attention can move among the dense and obvious aspects of the body, including anything from self-image to the feeling of bone and skin. We can also attend to the temperature of the body, the movement of breath within the body, feelings, and even subtle energetic movements. The mind-body is much like the layers of an onion; each layer of an onion can be seen as a pattern seemingly separate from the other layers, yet on closer inspection, the sheaths of an onion interpenetrate one another, each one contingent and provisional. The kośas represent the interconnection of mind, body, emotion, thought, and stillness—aspects of human experience that cannot ultimately be separated from one another.

Any type of stress, whether it's physical, mental, or emotional, causes tension in our bodies that accumulates from static, repetitive, or sustained posture. Posture can include physiological holding patterns, but according to the theory of the kośas, any postural holding pattern is both physiological and psychological.

The term *kośa* means "sheath," "cover," "subtle body," "treasury," or "lexicon," and comes from the root *kus,* meaning "to enfold." The sheaths are of five layers or frames that fold into one another. They consist of (1) *annamaya kośa,* the anatomical sheath, made up of bones, tendons, muscle groups, and other gross or dense masses; (2) *prāṇamaya kośa,* the physiological sheath, made up of the circulatory system including the respiratory, nervous, lymphatic, and immune systems; (3) *manomaya kośa,* the psychological sheath, which includes the mind, feelings, and the processes that organize experience; (4) *vijñanamaya kośa,* the frame responsible for intellect and wisdom; and (5) *ānandamaya kośa,* the aspect of the body where everything is as it should be, often described either as a sense in the body of everything being OK, or referred to as the sense of the body when one feels that the body is simply a form of energy or impersonal flow.

One cannot talk about one sheath without talking about the ways in which it is contingent upon other sheaths, because they all work together as a whole, an interdependent life cycle. When the breath draws in through the nostrils and my respiratory diaphragm descends, I feel the breath in terms of sensation, my mind conceives of the breath in terms of an image, name, or form, and if I am somewhat focused, I may also have thoughts about the breath, memories, or feelings associated with the simple activity of in-breathing. All of the sheaths work together, like a lexicon or matrix, and the theory of the kośas describes that interconnection.

The five kośas offer a prism through which we can observe, feel, and investigate the mind-body working as a whole. This is something that was described in great detail and in a different language by Sigmund Freud at the turn of twentieth century. Sometimes we forget that Freud was originally a physician, and that almost all of his first patients came to him with physical symptoms. Freud would have them lie down on a long couch with their eyes closed and describe with language what they were feeling in their bodies. He would sit in a chair behind his patients so as not to infringe on their psychic space. His startling discovery, in what would become the "talking cure," was that physical symptoms always had a psychological counterpart. As people would talk about their physical symptoms, the symptoms would move and, in some instances, pass away all together. Talking, or the psychological recognition of what was being felt in the body, brought mind and body together in a way that was healing.

To say that these symptoms were purely physiological would be incorrect, because through language, and what Freud later called free association, those symptoms changed. And to say that these holding patterns are purely psychological, or to go further and say that these patterns are all in the minds of those patients, would be incorrect, if only because the physical symptoms they presented were undeniable. In other words, no deep holding pattern in the mind-body is exclusively physical or exclusively psychological, but rather a combination of both.

What this means to the yoga practitioner is that one is always working both with mind and body, and to conceive of a yoga practice as purely a physiological form of exercise is to miss the internal and subtle aspects of yoga, which includes the psychological. So if we choose a particular aspect of the body, such as the myofascial system or the emotions or the nervous system or the breath, we see it against and within the backdrop of the other sheaths of the mind-body.

The annamaya and prāṇamaya kośas are the simplest layers to get a feel for. You can think of these sheaths as a three-dimensional matrix that connects every cell to every other cell within our entire body of bones, muscles, organs, and skin, all animated by the breath. Perhaps the most important quality of this sheath is that it records all physical, mental, emotional, and cognitive activity.

An example of how these two sheaths interconnect can be seen within the myofascial system, which is composed of collagen and elastin fibers, which provide flexibility and support for the entire musculoskeletal system, connecting all structures to other structures, forming a protective conduit to keep external pressure off the neurovascular system, and holding memory. All sheaths hold memory. It is of course not just the mind that maintains memory but the unconscious, which is normally associated with our psychology and exists primarily in the body.

What is most compelling about the kośas is that they offer us a paradigm through which we can feel and investigate the interpermeating nature of the mind, body, breath, and energy as it manifests in the here and now. I have found the kośas a transformational tool because they show how the interconnections between different organizing principles of human experience work together. The breath links up with changes in the mind, and the mind in turn affects our perception of the body in time and space, and our habitual patterns of movement influence and are influenced by all these other links in the chain. Posture affects perception, and perception affects posture. Furthermore these links are much more than separate knots or ties, because they are made up of one another. The mind and body are made up of magnitudes and dimensions, connections that are interwoven and inseparable.

This gets at the heart of yoga, namely insight into the very union, ecology, and interplay of life as it manifests in human form. Whether it's a strong sensation in the stomach or a daydream during a breathing practice, every aspect of human experience contains lines that tie back into one another. How can we posit any form of duality and separateness once we see just how fundamental are these interconnections?

I have always been so impressed by the teachings of B.K.S. Iyengar when he pulls together the striking connections between breathing, movement, and the mind. Very few yoga teachers have been able to move so thoroughly and deliberately through the precise techniques of yoga postures and breathing where suddenly the limb of āsana opens up to the other limbs. Practicing yoga postures with precision of attention cuts through any polarities in our thinking because the mind gets so focused on immediate experience that the experience opens into a wider dimension of interconnection.

The kind of attention subtle āsana practice requires focuses the mind on process rather than structure; change rather than stability, and flow rather than discrete movements. This opens up the mind to the present moment, the feeling of spontaneity, change, and chance, pulling the mind out of the duality of subject and object, mind and matter, submission or dominion, because yoga postures offer insight into the value of all forms of human experience, be they physical, mental, emotional, or perceptual. As we go deep into the matter of our bones we find not building blocks or pieces in conversation but rather a complicated web of relations between various parts of the whole. Yoga is synonymous with that whole. The universe of even one breath cycle is completely whole and unbroken. When the mind breaks things up into parts and pieces belonging to a "me," that whole is turned into fragmented experience. Yoga refers to the undivided wholeness and intimate interconnection of reality.

The body and mind that at first appear to the practitioner as solid structure eventually reveal themselves as constantly changing process, because any structure is, at base, process. Yoga is the practice of attending to this process. Another way of thinking about the interconnectedness of the mind and body, and of the kośas in particular, is through the myth of Indra's Net.

This Indian myth occurs in both Hinduism and Chinese Mahayana Buddhism. It conceives of the abode of Indra, the Hindu god of space, in which there is a net that stretches infinitely in all directions. At every intersection of the net there is a jewel so highly polished and perfect that it reflects every other jewel in the net. Each and every jewel in the web is intimately connected with every other jewel so that any change of pattern in the web is replicated throughout every sector and layer of its system. The entire net is interconnected and interdependent. When any jewel in the net is touched, all other jewels in any node are affected. This speaks to the hidden interconnectedness and interdependency of everything and everyone in the universe.

Returning to the example of fascia in the annamaya sheath, the collagen and elastin fibers make the sheath of fascia flexible and strong. In addition, the elastin gives muscles elasticity and flexibility, while the collagen provides stability. Whether in body or mind, we always find elasticity and structure, pliability and inertia. In the body and mind, we find dynamic stability, which refers to the way these five sheaths create a sense of structure yet are constantly in motion as well as states of regeneration. At one level something seems fixed in a pattern, and if you look a little deeper, you will find motion. Keep looking into motion and you will again find form. We are always dancing between form and impermanence. As an example, collagen, which is a moving aspect of the fascia, also supports the musculoskeletal structure. Efficiency and function of all body systems and movements, including the relationship between the connective tissue and muscle, depends on the balance within the myofascial system. And of course the myofascial system is also in a state of balance with the emotional body that is also interdependent with the nervous system, immune system, and mind. In other words, we see in the theory of the five sheaths an ecology of interdependence. This ecological, physiological, and psychological approach to the mind-body allows us to see contingency at work. Parts work together, and within parts we find subcycles supported by other subcycles ad infinitum.

Like the net of Indra, the theory of the kośas shoots holes in the assumption or imputation of a solid and fixed universe "out there." The capacity of one jewel to reflect the light of another jewel from the other edge of infinity is something that is difficult for the linear mind to comprehend. The fact that all nodes are simply reflections indicates that there is no particular single source point from whence it all arises. Our experience of body occurs through feeling, mind, and perception, and the ability to perceive rests on a body and sense organs that act as media through which the data of perception flows.

Furthermore, the fact that all nodes are simply a reflection of all others implies the illusory nature of all appearances. Appearances are thus not reality but a reflection of reality. If all the kośas are like threads of a web, and the unique patterns within each aspect of a human being weaves within the kośas, one cannot continue to practice even the physical aspects of yoga postures without at the same time recognizing the psychological and relational aspects of practice as well.

Even mind and consciousness, as categorized in the third kośa, manomaya kośa, the psychological sheath, which includes the mind, feelings, and the processes that organize experience as well as the fourth kośa, vijñanamaya kośa, the frame responsible for intellect and wisdom, are interconnected.

The final layer of the mind-body is the kośa of ānanda. Ānanda is the felt sense in mind and body that everything is OK just the way it is. Ānanda is the embodiment, even momentarily, of contentment. It's much like the feeling of tuning into the breath, even if it is stirred up, and feeling that one part of the breath that is completely relaxed, no matter how small. The term *ānanda* comes from the verbal root *nand,* which means "to rejoice." Ānandamaya kośa is the sheath that represents the joy in stillness. Unlike the outer sheaths of muscles or the inner sheaths of emotional patterns and thought, the innermost sheath of ānandamaya kośa is the sheath of perfection. It is similar to the Tantric descriptions of the middle axis of the body—*suṣumnā nāḍī,* which is empty and stainless, like the blue flute played by Kṛṣṇa at Vṛndivan.

Ānandamaya kośa describes the nature of pure awareness, which is empty and without the substance of self. It is the selfless self. It is clear and unpolluted, free from avarice and cultural impressions. It can't even be recognized as a thing unto itself. Much like the experience of *mūla bandha* or insight into emptiness, it is untouched. It is free from binding and coming apart, gaining and losing, coming and going. It is interdependent with the other sheaths and always demonstrates the point of stillness around which the other sheaths vibrate. It is the experience of simple awareness uncluttered by the fluctuations of the mind, even though it is part of that which fluctuates (*prakṛti*).

Ānandamaya kośa is the experience of awareness free of grasping. It is the mind and body without artifice. Without any special techniques, one can feel this standing still. The posture *samstitihi* literally means "to stand with equal balance." It refers to the balanced interrelation of the five kośas. The emotional body, nervous system, breath, mind, and heart are all in balance with one another.

The tendency of restriction in one sheath to transmit dysfunction to other parts is accounted for by the ways in which the kośas interpenetrate one another. You can also talk about the replication of patterns within the body as a characteristic of fascia and the nature of the whole fascial system.

As long as we are breathing, as long as our fluids are circulating, old structure is being demolished and removed while new material is being imported and built into new body parts. The body is not perfectly still;

it is always in dynamic motion. The mind is a changing process as well. But the motion has a sense of stability to it when the sheaths are in balance. Our electrical and chemical systems are constantly informing one another of, and responding to, the latest developments and needs. In addition to these routine processes of renewal and repair there are exceptional items that need taking care of from time to time. Some of these exceptional items we will be aware of, such as a minor cut, a sensitive hamstring, or an insect bite. Others will escape our attention provided we are healthy. One of the qualities of good health is the ability of our self-healing mechanism to take care of an endless list of minor imbalances and repairs without the need to divert our attention. Provided we don't overload our systems, we have the flexibility to accommodate a whole variety of stressors. It is only when our system loses flexibility that we start running the risk of deteriorating health, when problems that should be temporary tend to hang on or become chronic, or we may become very sensitive to substances or energetic influences that would not trouble a healthy person.

Think about inflexibility in psychological terms as well. When the mind is unable to hold several viewpoints simultaneously, when it is impossible to listen in a conversation, or when we find ourselves clinging to one perspective, we are caught in inflexibility. It is not just the body that becomes more flexible in yoga postures, but the mind as well. And when the mind is inflexible, those mental states are usually accompanied by or give rise to strong emotions. In moments of anger, jealousy, greed, or envy, we find ourselves clinging to a singular viewpoint at the expense of any other perspective. The mind moves in grooves with qualities similar to those of a stiff arm bone in a shoulder socket—tightness, discomfort, and stress.

The kośas operate within a global ecosystem of mind/body/ecology. In the larger system of the mind-body, what sorts of things happen to us that reduce our flexibility to renew and repair routinely? In the contemporary science of systems theory, it is said that a healthy system is one that knows how to repair itself. This is called "robustness." Robustness refers not just to the strength of a system but also to its ability to repair itself. In interdependence, the kośas influence and account for all of our bodily processes. If one part of the body loses its flexibility, it tends to break down often. A system that breaks down often educates itself by becoming stronger through flexibility. This is where the qualities and functions of the fascial system really start to account for themselves. Fascia has great flexibility and is fundamentally influential in all of our bodily processes. If a fascia in one part of the body loses its flexibility due to mechanical inhibition or a toxic or malnourished environment, it may affect any other part or system. Similarly, kośa restriction can be of an emotional nature as well. Thus, the five kośas account for the web or matrix that keeps all of the systems of the body communicating with one another.

Deepen the breath, with immediate attention, and stay with the breath for a little longer, and all sorts of movements may start. Emotion may start to surface, and held-in emotion is yet another cause of reduced flexibility. Even the mere alteration of thought or attention can facilitate flexible movement. Attitude and intention of the practitioner create an atmosphere where a holding pattern feels secure enough to risk the possibility of letting go. As the breath moves, the mind moves; as the mind moves, the nervous system moves; and you cannot separate the movements of mind, breath, and body any more than you can take the essence "onion" out of any layer of an onion. Yoga is the node where at least two things meet, and we find such nodes wherever the sheaths come together. But the sheaths are always together, and that is the great paradox: mind and body are always working with breath in the same way that the present moment is always occurring whether you are there for it or not.

The elastic nature of the kośas enables them to carry the memory or intelligence of exactly how the body would like to be arranged to enjoy the greatest ease. Every symptom is an attempt at arranging the sheaths of the mind-body in such a way that balance can be regained. Sheaths of the body under tension are always trying to pull the body back to this state of greatest ease. All psychological symptoms, whether anxiety, depression, or even emotional pain, are the psyche's attempt to balance the sheaths of the mind-body process. Although many symptoms do not at first seem to have a purpose, they are almost always attempts at balance, no matter how perverted. The breath and the body know in full detail and with total accuracy exactly what they need to do, and what assistance they need in order to return to a state of ease.

The kośas teach us that the systems of the human mind and body, like the larger systems in ecology, are open to, and interact with, their environments, and that they can acquire qualitatively new properties throughout their life cycle, resulting in continual evolution. In other words, we are extremely elastic, and what appears on the surface as fixed and closed is actually an impermanent and flexible process. Rather than reducing an entity such as the human mind or body to the properties of its parts or elements (for example, organs or cells), kośa theory focuses on the arrangement of and relations between the parts, which connect them into a whole. In the Vedas, the relationships between the kośas are not just considered in terms of layers but are also thought of as food for one another. The kośas nourish one another.

We are so used to categorizing the body into parts or looking at our psychological symptoms as somehow separate from the rest of our life. Or we practice the physically demanding practices of Hatha Yoga without opening up to the way these practices affect other aspects of our lives. But whatever we are engaged in is part of a larger system. This is the teaching of Indra's Net. The nature of the mind-body is a whole system and so, just like an economy, a family, a company, a community, and many other things, can be looked at as interdependent systems.

Yoga challenges us to take a view that would include all the factors involved in any given situation and examine how they relate to one another as well as how they work as a whole. This requires flexibility of perspective and focused attention. To deal with a whole system, we can't leave anything out as irrelevant.

The systems of the body are dynamic; they change, move, and develop. Frozen pictures of how things are supposed to be do us no good; we need to deal with live systems, whatever surprising directions that might take us in. This is what we call "beginner's mind."

The attitude of a beginner allows us to pay attention to the interactivity of not only the subtle elements of the body or the breath in a movement but also to all eight limbs of practice. Nonviolence, for example, begins in your own breath and extends out through your body and into relationship with the interdependent system of which you are only a part.

# 12. Working with the *Kośas*

THE BREATH WRAPS itself like ribbons around the internal structure of the body. It wraps but does not bind. It moves but does not stick. It's only the mind that sticks. As easily as the breath enters the body and mind, it leaves. But the body and mind are dependent on the breath. We only know the feel of the body because of the breath. Take this a step further: If there were no breath, there would be no body to know.

The breath animates the web of life, and in human form this is most effortlessly experienced as breathing. Physiologically, the heart pumps our blood, but the larger organs, including the stomach and spleen, liver and kidneys, are sewn to the respiratory diaphragm—a perfect location. The pumping and vibrating of the major organs of the body occur through the movement of the respiratory diaphragm.

An interesting function of human physiology is that the respiratory diaphragm also controls the nervous system. The respiratory diaphragm, in its movements up and down, like a wave rising and descending, controls the rhythm of the nervous system particularly in the thoracic spine. In fact, in yoga's model of the physiology of the nervous system, it is said that the nervous system primarily originates in the thoracic spine at the same location that the respiratory diaphragm hooks into the thoracic vertebrae. This would be somewhere close to the twelfth thoracic vertebra.

The breath presses the nervous system into rhythm and as such spreads out across the body like waves on the cosmic ocean or roots beneath the surface of the earth. A root structure, a wave pattern, or even the web of a spider is a combination of lines and circles with an organic purpose. The mind and breath interweave just like patterns throughout the vegetable kingdom, as can be seen in the branching of nerves, blood vessels, and other physiological systems. The One becomes the many as organic complexity evolves.

Like the mind that either spreads out or gets concentrated, like water in a river that diverts and meets up again, the breath, too, moves from the one to the many, from singularity to infinity. When the sensation of the breath is felt in the nostrils, it occurs first as a fine and singular line, a thread, a simple stream coursing through the nostrils. Then it spreads, beginning at the root of the palette where the tongue becomes the throat. It drifts across the shoulder blades and spreads the collarbones away from each other. The inhalation continues as a widening movement across the rib cage, and with close attention one can feel all the bones in the body rotating externally during the inhale and internally during the exhale.

Exhaling pulls the ribs close together and inhaling spreads them out again, drawing the wings of the kidneys across the back, wrapping the skin around the side ribs and pulling toward the front midline of the torso.

With awareness and concentration we can not only follow the patterning of the breath but also control it. In mindfulness of the breath we watch the breath closely without interfering with it. We learn about its structure and patterning as well as its impermanence. But in prāṇāyāma and āsana, we manipulate the breath. In prāṇāyāma we stretch the breath, as Richard Freeman says, "like the sun stretches light." Without stretching the breath throughout the five sheaths of the body, it moves in habituated patterns. Likewise, when we stretch the breath, the mind that follows the breath is stretched into longer and longer spans of attention until the mind itself—the seemingly solid, stable mind—dissolves into a stream of momentary perceptions arising and passing away, moment to moment, coming from nowhere and going nowhere, yet continuing in sequence without pause. The breath, too, arises and falls away, revealing the mind and breath as a singular phenomenon, which has the effect for the practitioner of placing him or her in a nondual state of awareness.

Most of the confusion about the teaching of the kośas occurs when it is assumed that the kośas refer only to the physicality of the body. It is easy to fall prey to the pull of a Judeo-Christian cultural attitude of a mind split from the body. If we superimpose mind over body on the kośa system, it seems like there is a mind that stands outside these five layers of body. But the kośa theory is the antidote to the mind-body split because it includes the mind within its sheaths. The kośas describe a whole human being rather than a mind apart from the layers of the body alone. One cannot make a case for the workings of the mind alone or for the priority consciousness has in any given moment, because mind, breath, body, and stillness are of one piece, and if the kośas are truly interdependent, one aspect cannot operate without interactions with all the others.

If mind is treated as something apart from the kośas, they become nothing more than an elaborate way of talking about "body and mind." But traditional texts make it quite clear that physicality refers to the entire range of material conditions both inside and outside our minds and bodies. It includes not only the sense organs but also their objects: colors and shapes, sounds, smells, tastes, tactile sensations, as well as such disparate things such as space, gender, heat, nutriment, decay, impermanence, and so on. The functioning, decay, and impermanence of the kośas allow us to see the "unfindability," in the mind and body, of a stable and sustaining self. On close investigation a picture emerges of a seamless, dynamic process of experience, where not only the body-mind split but also the subject-object split is dissolved. Learning to experience things in terms of these five kośas erodes our sense of being "a mind inside a body inside a world."

The kośas are not something surrounding or happening to "me."

Where is the "I" among these sheaths? When we try to find a solid "I" having experience within the frame of the kośas, it is impossible. Since the kośas interpenetrate one another in a seamless flow, if we posit permanence or something essential and lasting within that flow, it gets interrupted. This is experienced in mind and body as feeling blocked. Having configured "self," "mind," "body," and "world" as discrete things, we feel that each is cut off from the other, thus blocking the flow of life. This leads to degrees of alienation, in which we feel "out of touch" with our body, our emotions, other people, and the environment. There are moments in life—such as when we are one with the natural world, making love, playing with a child, creating art, ingesting psychotropic drugs, or sitting in meditation—when the blocks within the kośas are temporarily dissolved. But as soon as the mind comes in, or more specifically the "I"-making function of the mind (*ahaṇkāra*), the blocks return again, leading to feelings of separateness and alienation. However, we are not trapped in a destiny outside of our control, and it is the perspective of the kośas that guide us in seeing that all attempts to create permanence in a dazzling and unstable world will only bring separateness and discontent.

Our subjective experience always appears on the surface as a "me" having experience of some thing "inside" or "outside" a somewhat-stable self. Yoga practice shows us over and over again that what seems like an experience belonging to "me" is simply the contact of perception and stimulus. And the person that perceives, along with that which is perceived, is changing, unpredictable, and unstable. If I like what I experience, I try to repeat it (raga), and if I do not like it, I try to avert it (dveṣa), thus giving myself the feeling of being a real self.

When I feel a bone and create a theory that the leg bone is mine, I give substantiality both to what I perceive and to the self that is perceiving. However, these are simply kośas—in this case the first and third—coming into contact with each other. This contact is one moment in a seamless flow of changing and, paradoxically, impersonal conditions.

Most practitioners view the kośas as a convenient way of describing the interconnection of mind and body. However, the kośas are also a theoretical construct through which we can see the turning cycle of saṁsāra, conditioned existence. A separate self sets up the conditions for addiction, because all addictive patterns stem from the flip-flop back and forth between attachment, aversion, and the consequence of these two reactionary patterns, namely, feeling like a self.

Is there a self that inhabits this mind and body? How can we find it? How do we know it is there? Where is its location?

A personality or psychology convinced of the self as primary leads to a personality embedded in existential disorientation. Since feeling like a separate self solidifies both subject and object—"me" and what is either "outside" or "inside" me—one feels stuck in a compartmentalized world. But the kośas are not separate compartments. They are interpermeating forms moving about within and around one another. The more obsessively we cling to "self," the more we reinforce a compartmentalized perception of reality configured by existential confusion. The very insistence on being "someone" blocks the possibility of freedom in being no one. As soon as "someone" is born, the anguish of torment, grief, pain, depression, and anxiety is inevitable.[1]

After looking deeply into the nature and operation of the kośas, it no longer makes sense to commit to a reality or even continually construct a life where we insist on a self that exists independent of the kośas. This maintains the feeling of a self inside a mind inside a body inside a world. Any attempt to ensure the survival of a self inside a mind—strategies that are ingrained and deeply unconscious—create anxiousness and a self-centered mode of perception. Longing to be someone keeps us self-absorbed and intensifies the subject-object split.

Patañjali says that the mind and body and even awareness is *svarūpa śūnya* (empty of self-form). The word *śūnyatā* derives from the root *shu,* which interestingly enough means "swollen." Something swollen is something beyond original measure, boundless, and by definition, beyond fragmentation and compartmentalization. This is the heart of the kośa theory: by using the lens of these sheaths that make up mind and body, we begin to see that the sheaths, like the jewels in Indra's net, penetrate one another, are formed by one another, and though singular in one way, are from a larger view, part of everything else in existence.

There is nothing to cling to. Not holding on to any one thing, even the need to be a self, drops the yoga practitioner into a reality that is unmeasured. This unmeasured reality is the way that the mind-body process actually is: a seamless part of a changing whole. There is only consciousness and its objects appearing and disappearing, a moving gyroscope of mind, body, and world, forever impossible to disentangle from one another because they are made up of one another.

# 13. *Saṁskāras*

## WEBS OF MIND AND BODY

THE OFT-QUOTED SECOND line of the second chapter of the *Hatha Yoga Pradīpika* reminds us that when the breath moves through the body with agitation, the mind, too, becomes agitated; as the breath becomes still, so too does the mind. "When the breath is in motion the mind is in motion. The breath being without motion, the mind becomes motionless."[1] The breath, mind, and body work together, as they are inseparable.

In our exploration of the five kleṣas we have looked at the strategies we use, consciously and unconsciously, that cause us to contract around that which is unpleasant or impermanent in order to find some sure footing. This contracting, aversion, or pulling has profound psychological effects (the six poisons), which also replicate through the living body. In the last chapters we looked at how perception can pick up anything in the field of awareness and create a story about "me" out of it. Our misperception and misidentification with our experience is a great burden. Now we will look at how these patterns manifest energetically.

Rarely can our attention remain undivided to stay, for sustained periods, with the subtlety of breathing or the experience of silence. We are so accustomed to the innumerable complexities of living that we are largely unaware of the subtleties of breathing, the simplicity of awareness, the felt sense of the mind and body in stillness. This is one of the reasons we practice yoga postures. We practice postures to learn about waking up the intelligence of the body, and then we also cultivate the opposite: learning how to observe the body and mind while leaving both alone. Yoga practices are constructed quite differently in different schools and across different cultures, depending on what aspects are given more emphasis. Regardless of what limb, stage, or process one is pursuing as their chosen path, most paths share the same dance between stretching mind and body outside historical parameters and self-imposed narratives and then settling mind and body in complete stillness.

The term we use for "posture," *āsana,* literally means "to sit." Most scholars and practitioners translate *āsana* to refer to sitting in meditation or being in a meditative position such as *padmāsana* (Lotus pose) or *virāsana* (Hero's pose). In the context of Patañjali's *Yoga-Sutra,* however, we can contemplate this term in a more figurative sense as meaning "to sit with." A yoga posture is an opportunity to "sit with" what is arising from moment to moment with acceptance and patience, steadiness and ease. Patañjali states that the practice of āsana leads to the dissolution of duality, where the sense of "me" and "my body" dissolve into each other, leaving only felt experience but no sense of a separate self having the experience. Like the time of day when the coming of night and the conclusion of daylight collapse into each other, or swimming in perfect summer water where the difference between warm and cool are no difference at all, a movement is so fully executed that one is reduced to not even a word.

Contemplating āsana psychologically turns a yoga pose into a tool of awareness, an opportunity for liberation. It also broadens our understanding of āsana to include not just practicing headstand or back bend but also washing dishes, being present in relationship, walking, sleeping, and talking. Āsana can permeate the rest of our day, our entire life for that matter, and give us access to a more spacious sense of being. The form of the pose is secondary to what that pose is orienting the mind-body toward.

Since contemporary āsana practice is the most common door through which people come into contact with yoga, it is usually the first limb of practice. Whether or not this has always been the case is up for debate, especially since Indian historical material on the history of āsana is quite conjectural. In Sanskrit texts that describe āsana in more detail than Patañjali's *Yoga-Sutra,* we usually hear of a six-limbed practice that begins with āsana rather than the first two limbs of ethics. Even though there is no mention of ethics, āsana is always considered a practice that brings practitioners to the place of nonseparation.

For many of us, the movements of body and breath bring us into contact with habitual and often unconscious patterns of movement, thought, and feeling. When one first begins yoga practice, it takes only a short period of time to learn about the ways in which the body is conditioned: we can extend our hamstrings only so far, the breath is deeper on one side of the torso compared with the other, the spine is inflexible in certain motions, and the mind is distracted during certain parts of the breath cycle. Soon after recognizing our physical limits, we also notice how these limits give rise to preferences—we like poses that give us pleasure and lean away from postures that cause us difficulty. However, this difficulty is not just a physical limitation but also what the mind does with that limitation, and this is the crucial point: duḥkha is self-generated. Difficult sensation in the body is not necessarily a form of suffering; rather, it is what the mind adds to the experience that creates dissatisfaction and stress. For example, when deeper patterns of uncomfortable sensations build up in the body, say in the hips, the mind becomes impatient. Impatience is a sign that we are having a hard time staying present with sensations in the body. The sensations are acceptable as phenomenal experience, but the mind and emotions have preferences that arise alongside those sensations, creating a gap between what are actually arising as phenomena and what we are trying to do with those experiences. That gap is called duḥkha. The mind follows sensations in the body with preference, interpretation, and conceptualization, described by Patañjali as *citta vṛtti* (fluctuations of consciousness).

Āsana practice approached psychologically takes us right to the heart of sensations arising and passing as well as what the mind contracts around those sensations. It's a practice that cuts through the armor of preferences built into our psychophysical makeup. Yoga postures stretch us beyond these preferences. Since the body is always responsive, we move within its envelope in order to cultivate an unrehearsed immediacy of contact and knowing—action without dust.

Because different yoga poses set up various patterns of breathing and physiological action, postures are invitations into the psychological and physiological webs that form the matrix of the mind-body. Posture sequences open up different layers and movements of mind and body and thus work on the sheaths of mind and body in distinct ways. Traditional posture sequences create balance in the mind-body because postures complement one another and alternate between stretching and stilling the breath.

If we only practice poses that reinforce our zones of comfort, we end up with a yoga practice that moves prāṇa only in habitual ways. And if we are used to overexertion or hyperactivity, then the pranic patterns in the body will be reinforced in this way also. So finding the balance between steadiness and ease in yoga postures also requires playing with the limits of our physical sensibilities, because all of our sense organs are conditioned in habitual ways. Some habits are benign, while others are like archaic monuments in the body that we visit as tourists of our own self-image. The basic tendencies or grooves in both mind and body are called "saṁskāras." They influence the way we think and move, the way we act and breathe, and even the basic conditioning of the respiratory system, nervous system, immune function, and all of the subtle operating systems of the body.

We can also think of saṁskāras as latent impressions, predispositions, webs, imprints, inherent tendencies, molds, or internal grooves.

The term comes from *sam* (to come together) and *kr* (action). The term *saṁskāra* is interchangeable with the common Sanskrit term *vāsanā,* which also refers to predispositions from past impressions or actions. These karmic memory traces are primarily unconscious residue from previous experience. Every new moment contributes to these traces, like dust to velvet. Karma is like an accumulation of dust. In traditional Indian philosophy, these latent impressions that predispose the mind and body in specific ways are somewhat mysterious. In the meeting with Pattabhi Jois at Marpa House in Boulder, it was interesting the way he brushed off questions about alignment technique in yoga postures if he felt that the student was striving in an egoic way. If someone asked him how to achieve the next back-bend sequence, he would just say, "Next lifetime." This was a joke, but it also served as a way of setting ambition in context. He was much more interested in talking about the internal process of yoga than he was the physical details of postures, even though it was the subject of physicality that most students were asking about.

Physical practice is an internal process when we pay close attention to what the breath and mind are doing in any given moment. Saṁskāras, as conditioned patterns, influence the way we perceive and organize experience. And since anything that is conditioned is from the past, saṁskāras prevent a fresh meeting with the present moment because they inform the way that we meet, organize, filter, and elaborate upon that moment. The saṁskāras are like mental, emotional, and physical biases within the mind-body. The ongoing actions of body, speech, and mind that spring from the interaction of any given data with the habits of the saṁskāras reinforce the saṁskāras from moment to moment. This is the cause-and-effect model of karma as it operates in mind and body, making the saṁskāras psychophysical manifestations of karma.

The karmic effects in mind and body are like seeds that grow into particular modes of perception or particular ways of acting. Seeds that get planted over and over again are like habits that reinforce one another.

Thinking of the saṁskāras as bias is helpful because previous seeds prejudice in positive or negative ways the way we interact with succeeding moments. If we think of the poisons that Pattabhi Jois described—desire, anger, delusion, greed, envy, and sloth—as seeds, our unconscious habit of acting on those seeds reinforce those very energies. In relation to the saṁskāras, we can better understand the psychological and physical location of such seeds as conditioned patterns of mind and body. But if we also think of the saṁskāras as fields of consciousness, we can better understand how to work with both the saṁskāras and also the symptoms that manifest from their imbalance, because like any field, seeds germinate under certain conditions and don't come to fruition under others. Positive saṁskāras germinate based on positive mental states, and negative saṁskāras repeat in negative mental conditions. A shoulder moves within a certain spectrum of movement, and as we open up the shoulder joint, a new pattern of movement is formed. The saṁskāras are constantly evolving. Like a gardener working nonstop, our work is to cultivate the field of the saṁskāras in such a way that we monitor which karmic seeds evolve and in what way.

## *Context and Release*

The saṁskāras are like predispositions or contexts that the mind and body supply in each new moment of experience. When we have an experience, say of a sunset, we try to allow the sunset to reach us, to make an impression on us. But we tend to do that only by supplying a context within which we can receive the experience. We label the phenomenon as "sunset," compare it to other sunsets, and frame the experience in language. These contexts are fore-structures of understanding, preconceptions, or prejudices. We select contexts by choice: they are not given, and they are not built into the experience itself. A direct experience of a sunset, or the energetic flow of a posture, is inherently empty of conceptualizing, empty of meaning. Joseph Campbell says, "We are not trying to find the meaning in life but rather a deep experience of it." In fact, when we let go of the constant drive toward finding meaning, things become meaningful.

The process of experience, then, goes something like this: To begin with, a new experience enters us. It is without context. But because we know something about what the experience might be, based on preceding moments or past experience, we have a small collection of contexts that might be appropriate for whatever is going to arise. When the new data meets us, we take it in only partially, as it comes through the filters of the sense media and the mind. The sense organs and the mind quickly decide on the context that fits it best. The experience then seems completed by the context we give to it, but this is actually only a partial experience, because it is already an interpreted moment. Patañjali calls this *saṁyoga,* or the misapprehension of an experience in context with a fresh experience that has no context. Again, context is not "built in to experience."

On first consideration, having an experience of a sunset or a yoga posture or even another person without creating a context seems impossible. How are we to vacate prior experiences in order to have a fresh one? This is the psychological conundrum that Patañjali points out in his description of āsana. The problem is that we base our sense of self on these past experiences and filter all new information through that previously determined sense of self. How can something be experienced if the condition for the experience is to have already understood what it is about? This is a paradox, because nothing is more invisible than the next moment. In that case, all we have is this moment, which is without context—the context is an addition.

The way through this paradox is to recognize that we always shape our experience, mostly unconsciously, with the grooves of the mind-body, which in turn reinforce themselves, because the more that the mind and breath flow through conditioned grooves, the deeper those grooves become. When we are in a deep groove, it is hard to see a way out, or sometimes to even know that we are actually in a groove. However, when we begin to learn about our conditioning, we can see these patterns and how they limit our experience. Then we can be open to the alteration of these grooves that the present moment requires of us. Discovery is always a process of redefinition.

# 14. *Prāṇa*

## ENERGETIC FLOW

*PRĀṆA* IS a mysterious term, most commonly applied to the act of breathing. But it actually refers to something much more universal, traditionally describing life energy as a whole and the way energy vibrates, circulates, and forges new pathways. Prāṇa is the energy that animates life, and in human form prāṇa is most perceptible as the breath. When we go even farther into the breath itself, we see that it is made up of an infinite number of qualities, called *vāyuu*s, or "winds" of the breath. Like a full-color spectrum, there are many layers to the breath, with currents and subcurrents, texture and weave, and as one follows, feels, and gets to know the breath as a form of devotional practice, the breath reveals its many winds.

The winds are like currents of energy, and when we tune in to the various currents, we see they are made up of perception, thought, nervous system, cognition, and all activities of mind and body. Yoga practitioners, when sensitive to the internal currents of the body, use these currents to gather information about the functioning of mind and body. These winds of prāṇa are the fundamental processes of human existence. Energetic sensing brings us into contact with the subtle winds that move within us and govern perception and action.

Prāṇa, which we can translate as "life energy" or "breath," flows within meridians that spread throughout the body, and these meridians in turn are conditioned by the saṁskāras. Saṁskāras are internal structures that inform the way in which prāṇa flows through the mind-body and therefore the way we perceive, move, think, and act. Where do these habitual grooves come from? In most lineages, it is thought that these basic grooves come from three sources: nature, nurture, and past lives. *Nature* refers to the biological blueprint that we come into the world with. *Nurture* refers to the way in which that blueprint is formed in its meeting with environment and culture. *Past lives* is an essential category, because not all patterns in mind and body fit neatly into the two-category system of nature and nurture. Robert Wright, author of *The Moral Animal,* describes this well:

> Of course, you can argue with the proposition that all we are is . . . genes and environment. You can insist that there's . . . something more. But if you try to visualize the form this something would take, or articulate it clearly, you'll find the task impossible, for any force that is not in the genes or the environment is outside physical reality, as we perceive it. It's beyond scientific discourse . . . this doesn't mean it doesn't exist.[1]

Whether you believe in past lives or not (a future discussion to be sure), we must create an extra category for certain tendencies that are unexplained via nature or nurture.

The practice of yoga postures invites us into this domain between—literally right in between—the psychological and physiological components of conditioned existence. As you can see from investigation of the saṁskāras, you cannot talk about a psychological holding pattern without talking about physiology, and you can't explore physical holding patterns without looking at psychological grooves, because every saṁskāra is composed of and manifests the mental, emotional, energetic, and physical elements that make up the matrix of the mind-body.

Notice in yoga postures how certain physical sensations bring with them specific mental formations and emotions. The more we start thinking, the more agitated we become. Past impressions, associations, and memories are always lying dormant alongside physical sensations. History is always falling in our lap. To attend to the truth of what is happening, to the immediacy of our experience rather than to our ideas about what is happening, teaches us how to handle the events of experience with more clarity.

We live in a culture that tries endlessly to find more and more pleasure, thinking that sensory gratification in every sense organ will lead to happiness. We end up caught in numerous shopping options, consumers of instant gratification. The effect psychologically and physically is not only restlessness but also a mind and sense organs that are clogged up with sensory overload and the inability to take in anything with clarity. Life becomes about producing and consuming. So just beginning with simple movements and breathing, we return the mind-body to a less chaotic pace, and then, sense organ by sense organ, open up the channels, and eventually the heart, so that our perceptual faculties are less polluted. Then we can breathe again. Then we can be silent. And everything is crafted out of silence.

The inhale is born out of silence and the exhale returns us to silence. Thoughts and sensations arise and pass away to nowhere. Or is it everywhere? I always begin sitting meditation, āsana practice, and also prāṇāyāma by sitting silently and feeling the sense of body and breath occurring without interference. It's hard not to interfere. No longer offering mind and body to ceaseless distractions, they settle themselves by being left alone, like the noiseless flight of birds.

The practice of yoga postures is a practice of prāṇāyāma; both are rituals of attention animated by the currents of the breath. Āsana and prāṇāyāma practice have to do with following the flow of the breath and the flow of energy within the body. Once some concentration and ease is established, we notice where energy flows and where it is interrupted. We give immediate attention to the patterns and disruptions of the breath, the nervous system, the heart rate, and the feeling tone in the muscles, fascia, and so on. All of these objects of awareness become objects of meditation (*dhāraṇā*) and eventually opportunities for absorption (*dhyāna*).

As we deepen our focus on the quality of breath as it moves through the constantly changing configuration of mind-body, we come to see that there are two streams we are working with: a stream of breathing and a stream of mental formations. These two streams can be thought of as prāṇa (breath, life energy) and citta (mind, imagination, perception). We are trying to bring these two streams closer and closer together. The paradox is that the two streams are fundamentally intertwined, but our distracted mind keeps pulling them apart. The material and mental are two aspects of the same movement.

Yoga postures teach us how to perceive with ever greater levels of clarity. At first we breathe in, synchronizing the mind, body, and breath, then we breathe out. Eventually we begin to feel and even intuit dozens, if not hundreds, of universes in the breath. With clarity of attention, any feelings that arise, even if unpleasant, do not automatically become moments of dissatisfaction, nor do they unfold into stories of "me." Human experience is always carving out a world through limited means of perception, but it is precisely our limited means that open us up to the world. When we notice our drifting attention span or contraction in a shoulder socket, we at once notice our limited mobility and awareness and also pave a path out of the conditioning simply by bringing awareness to it. Remember that Pattabhi Jois did not go into details about how to work with the six poisons. Instead he treated them as symptoms and said, in fewer words, that if one wants to work with the symptoms of duḥkha, one begins not with the symptom itself but the five kleṣas and how they interact with one another in sequence.

In reflecting on Pattabhi Jois's suggestion, I have come to see the wisdom in witnessing the underlying patterns of attachment and aversion that give rise to a symptom rather than pursuing the elimination of the symptom itself. Our task is to move through the symptom toward the factors that give rise to the symptom in the first place.

Even on a collective level, greed, anxiety, depression, and even anger are not dealt with appropriately when we are quick to eliminate them from awareness. Anxiety in a culture often points to where change needs to happen; so in a collective sense, anxiety as a symptom is not something to eliminate too quickly. Likewise, painful sensation often teaches us the difference between feeling and reaction to feeling and is an inevitable part of human aging. Fear is important—an animal without fear is a dead animal. We shouldn't be too quick to eliminate the symptom; instead we try to get to the bottom of it. The process of *nirodha* is one of freeing obstructions, making space, getting to the bottom of things. *Nirodha* comes into English literally as "root," "radish," or "radical," which connote getting to the bottom of something. For Pattabhi Jois, the kleṣas bring us to the root cause of a symptom. This serves to map out the landscape of lived experience, which, when seen through the lens of the kleṣas, is seen to be always a constructed experience. This is a phenomenologically based psychology. Instead of starting with a diagnosis or even a creation myth, there is no context given in which everything is settled. Even when we do finally accept or let go of something, we don't always have an explanation for why or how it came to be in the first place. That is why we begin in the body. We begin our investigation of the symptoms of anguish, torment, and dissatisfaction by asking, What is it that is present in human experience in the present moment?

If yoga is the science of studying the way we perceive and construct our experience in order to bring about a fundamental shift in perception, we need to begin by understanding just how knowing operates. The way we know anything is not independent of the body, so waking up our pathways of perception means waking up the intelligence of mind and body. Not only do we have personal habits in the way we construct our world, we of course have personal habits of movement in the body. If the practice of Hatha Yoga is internally focused on these layers of mind and body, we come to study the way we know what we know and how intimately linked are our ways of knowing and ways of moving. Formal practice matures as awareness interiorizes, not through constant attention to superficial form. Otherwise, āsana practice becomes another field in which we act out the habitual demands of an unconscious self.

Many contemporary yoga communities find this out the hard way. People begin āsana practice who are drawn to the physical, aesthetic, and great benefits of the practice and there is nothing wrong with that; but when we lock on to a technique as the mode of improving our practice, the practice has the inverse effect. After a time, people do the practice, which consists of nothing other than the refinement of technique. The technique becomes confused with the experience of yoga, to say nothing of the other limbs, much like being a virtuoso musician who has no experience, no character, and no soul. Teachers and students of yoga may indeed have authentic openings, but from the perspective of an eight-limbed practice, there is work to do on many fronts. Practice must infiltrate everything, awareness capturing all of life, without exception. The breath is seen to be the morning wind; our ideas, the greening of a landscape; compassion, the embodied realization of our practice.

The habits of attachment and self-centeredness are relentless, and unless we continue to practice and move always beyond our favorite techniques, the habitual patterns of mind and body will continue to act themselves out. Then we come back to practice with more wisdom, because we can see technique as something instrumental much like the way a trumpet is used for manipulating sound but is not the source of sound itself.

When we go deep inside the sound of the breath as a whole, or when we listen carefully to the variations of the inhalation and exhalation, we are looking directly into the nature of the universe as it presents itself in these particular instances of experience. Feeling the subtle movements of the breath in the body and listening to these movements year after year has taught me how to pay attention to the way that the arising and passing of everything that moves through awareness happens and will continue to happen in a seamless flow. It has also taught me to view the world in terms of universal changes of events and processes. The breath is an integral part of the web of life, and studying the breath without being apart from it puts me in that very web. I am nothing other than the web of life.

When I transcend the habits of dualism and fragmentation, it's as if I become what I am observing. What is left for us to compare ourselves to? I feel the breath so clearly in the pelvic floor that the whole experience opens up before me and I experience what is occurring as a process of nature, the movement of butterfly wings, an ongoing linking of form and formlessness. The best way to describe this is as intimacy with the flow of all existence, in which the body and mind become unsurveyable, not apart from anything. When my mind finally settles into the full flow of the breath, it feels as if this is the ultimate purpose for being in the world. Nothing is clearer.

# 15. Body in Mind

HOW DO WE INTERRUPT the distracted and overly conceptual tendency of the mind in order to get concentrated? First of all, the spiritual practice of yoga is a journey of letting go, so it is important to always reconsider what it is that we are letting go of.

Posture practice is a way of noticing our tendency toward attachment (raga) and aversion (dveṣa) that cause us to repeat the patterns of not seeing things as they are (avidyā). All of our problems and feelings of dissatisfaction and suffering are caused by fixation and clinging—latching on to things and not being able to release them. This latching is a form of distraction, and it occurs within all of the sense organs (eyes, ear, nose, tongue, skin, and mind). We latch on to sound, form, feeling, thoughts, and perception.

The first step in the process of releasing these patterns of distraction occurs as we experience the body and mind as process rather than a substance. A yoga posture is a wonderful way of feeling things as they are through direct contact with energy flow. We notice how certain patterns of energy are difficult to stay with, and with patience and immediate awareness we stay with them. Learning to stay focused is effectively a process of learning to be free, because when we let go of something, we become free of it.

Letting go in the practice of yoga postures occurs when there is enough concentration present that we can slip into the flow of conditions that we call "yoga posture." A posture is a label we place on an experience of form, but beyond that label, the form reveals itself organically. For example, when you learn new alignment techniques in yoga postures, can you explore the difference between feeling new instruction from the inside out, or do you tend to superimpose a new image onto the body from the outside in?

Whatever factors we notice in the body, we see them as existing contingently on the way we perceive. Patañjali describes āsana practice as a tool for liberating the kleṣa activities, and the Tantric traditions, most notably the *Hatha Yoga Pradīpika,* describe āsana as a means of liberating the practitioner by seeing the nonduality of mind and body. This nonduality occurs in both traditions when the mind and breath become still enough to actually see that they are two sides of the same coin. Furthermore, since perception, breath, and body are always breaking up, and continually fluctuate together, we cannot pin our stories of reality on any of them. Whatever expectation we lay on our experiences—wanting this to turn out in previously determined ways—is always bound to come apart when the mind, breath, and body change. If the mind, breath, and body are eternally changing, and if we can barely define their location or existence, they cannot be taken as self; then letting go occurs naturally because it is the only option when clinging has failed. Raga and dveṣa come to an end when we see that the mind, breath, and body, as well as all objects of awareness (*ālambana*) are boundless, ownerless, and lacking inherent substantiality, coming and going contingent on conditions that likewise come and go.

When we give up our notions and labels of yoga postures, we relinquish our fixation on the reification of concepts: posture, body, leg, arm, bone, and so on. Experience no longer has to be "this" or "that." Thinking of "this or "that" binds us to a particular mode of existence that is conceptual and built on linguistic association and memory rather than on contact with real things. Patañjali warns of this in one the opening paragraphs of the *Yoga-Sutra,* where he states, "*Śabda-jñānānupāti vastu-śūnyo vilkapaḥ* (Conceptualization derives from linguistic knowledge, not contact with real things)."[1]

Notice how the word *śūnya* (empty) appears here to denote that the substance or object that we are aware of is empty of the linguistic and conceptual scaffolding that we construct around it. Emptiness is so hard to describe in words, not because it so sophisticated or subtle but precisely because it is so simple and basic to our nature. Often what is closest to us is what we have the hardest time noticing.

What Patañjali is saying here in reference to the body is that we tend to experience the body as a fabrication or concept. We look down below our hips and say, "leg," "thigh," "knee," and "foot." These labels give us the feeling that there is something there—a thing—and that based on this concept, we cling to the sense that something is truly there. Concepts, Patañjali suggests, have no real existence of their own, as they are empty of self-form (svarūpa śūnya). Even disposition is a malleable construction; nothing is cast in stone.

Concepts exist in our minds. So we are careful not to stop at the level of concept and to move forward in the direction of concentration beyond linguistic knowledge. We are so used to relating to our ideas of body and concepts of being in the body that sometimes we confuse our relationship with the concept as relationship with the body. But concept and embodiment are not the same thing.

Take for instance the notion that our body actually exists in the mind. When I first started practicing yoga, the teacher was fond of saying that my body is all in my mind. This seemed ridiculous at first, as I had feelings in my body that seemed independent from my thoughts. But then I began to discover, especially during intense āsana practice, there are certain sensations that we can allow ourselves to feel and others that, when they occur, we get out of there as fast as possible. Growing up as we do in our culture, the body is used to sitting in a chair, and thus we have tight hips, the femur bones don't rotate as they should, and the belly falls into the pubic bone. So when we begin practicing hip-opening poses, as a common example, we are brought into contact with sensations that we are not used to feeling, and those sensations have corresponding emotions and thought trains: one thought links up with another and another and another. This is where we often get distracted, because thoughts are glued to one another with memory, association, and habit. We get stuck in an idea: "There is sensation in leg. I do not like it. My leg hurts. I need to move. I am not flexible. Will I always be like this? The person next to me is so flexible. I am not good at anything. . . ."

I once had a teacher who would always come from across the room and adjust me during *kapotāsana* (Pigeon pose)—a pose that brought up a great deal of tension both in my hip flexors and in my mind. She would lean over and say, "Your body is in your mind, Michael." I would close my eyes and take a deep breath and refocus. Slowly I began to see that my experience of the body was made up of my ideas about the body and that when my ideas about my body were challenged, I was not present at all, just lost in preferences and stories. The well-timed words of this teacher created a shock to the ahaṇkāra—the "I"-maker, which I am fond of translating as "the storyteller." This temporarily paralyzed the self-continuity of the narrative of "I like" and "I don't like" and opened up a space of spontaneity. I can also characterize this space as creative and immediate awareness, because when our stories of how things should be are suspended, how things are come to light.

I still use these shock tactics, both while I practice and while I teach, and while they do not in themselves provide a final crossover into the territory of nirodha, they do provide a brief and immediate glimpse into unconditioned awareness, which we can call "the present moment." This is because all perceptions are misperception by virtue of our conditioning. This is not to say that perception is wrong or that misperception is bad, but that bolting down an idea doesn't serve the process nor does it serve the boundlessness of reality. Sometimes when practicing on my own, I use techniques to help interrupt the ongoing conversation of "me" that I normally call "thinking." One of these methods is asking the question, who is breathing? or who is moving? Relating to the body is like a dance, and it takes time before our awareness is focused enough to arrive fully in any given movement. The body has its own intelligence, as does the breath, so yoga postures teach us to let the thinking and conceptual mind give back to the body what is naturally in the body's domain.

What keeps us out of the body is thinking of ourselves as selves—as the central players around whom thoughts, feelings, and movements pivot. But since no thing has any inherent, essential, or abiding nature, there is really nothing that separates us from our bodies or each other. Every barrier is one we create through storytelling. We are not independent, separately locatable beings moving through an objective world, but rather unknowable, all-pervasive, and interconnected unknowables. We exist here and nowhere. Who practices yoga postures? Who breathes? Interrupting the linguistic narrative that accompanies almost all experience occurs when we can let go of clinging to ideas and get concentrated in action. This concentration leads to absorption, where action occurs but there is no sense of a "me" taking action. A posture is practiced simply for the sake of the posture. Yoga practice is not about true and false, inside or outside—it just means waking up to the inherent interconnectedness of reality, which is clear when one is clear.

You can see the arising of the story of self, born out of clinging to sensations in the body as mine, and watch the whole process without jumping out of it. If you look at experience, such a small percentage of it is either painful or pleasant—most is actually fairly neutral. It's the neutral, plain, common moments of experience that we also want to tune in to—stepping, lifting an arm, feeling a breath, and tilting the gaze. It is hard to stay in neutral feeling tones, especially in such an entertainment-based culture. Moving the body and being present in intentional movement teaches us how to receive experience on its own terms. Otherwise, what is this practice in service of?

When you see all of these thoughts about body and self just as thoughts about body and self, they lose their potency. When you see a pattern clearly, it loses its dynamic force. It is almost like looking into another person's eyes. You look into the eyes of another and the mind fills with all of kinds of ideas and emotions. It's hard to hold the gaze. But when the minds stops running away creating stories, then you just release the averting gaze back into the still gaze, and then you can see and also be seen. Likewise, when we recognize a pattern as a pattern, we release it simply by the fact that it has been seen. "Seeing" denotes that it doesn't have a grip on us anymore because there is increased space. This space, called "nirodha," is much like a force field or a creative energy that is born when the *vṛtti* is seen as it is; much like when you let go of a habitual addiction, you now have more energy for new endeavors because you are no longer bound by repetitive and unconscious patterns. As we push or hold on, we create a self—a structure or edifice that makes us feel embedded in something. But the self is not unified—like the breath, it comes and goes with experience. Perhaps we are verbs rather than nouns.

# 16. Letting Go

## *ĀSANA* AND MEDITATION INTERTWINED

HOW DO WE GO beyond likes and dislikes, beyond the dichotomies our minds are always creating? We do so by letting go of clinging, even the subtle clinging to ideas of self. When we lose the sense of a separate self that comes with habits and preferences, we become one with everything. We practice Serpent (*bhujaṅga*) and we become a serpent. We practice Eagle (*garuḍa*) and we become an eagle. We practice Heron pose (*kraunca*) and we become a heron. We practice in full connection with the earth (*pṛthvī*) and we become earth. When we let go, the non-dual, united nature that we call "yoga" comes forth correcting the waywardness of our distractions and misperceptions. In the realization of a holistic and integrated reality, of which we are only a part, sensitivity, devotion, and love burst forth.

> "Fetch me from over there a fruit of the Nyagrodha tree."
>
> "Here is one, sir."
>
> "Break it."
>
> "It is broken, sir."
>
> "What do you see there?"
>
> "The seeds, almost infinitesimal."
>
> "Break one of them!"
>
> "It is broken, sir."

> "What do you see?"
>
> "Nothing, sir."
>
> The father said: "My son, that subtle essence which you do not perceive there, of that very essence this great Nyagrodha tree exists. Believe it, my son, that that is the subtle essence—in that all things have their existence. That is the truth. That is the self. And you, Svetaketu, you are that."[1]

This exercise in nondual teaching comes from the *Chāndogya Upaniṣad.* It is only the grooves of perception and our accompanying concepts that keep us from being eagles, herons, trees, or ocean tides. Yoga returns us to spontaneous meditation, which is actually a nonmeditation, moving us even beyond technique. In other words we are not trying to meditate or even trying to practice. We are tuning in to the naturally existing sate of meditation, which is full engagement with what actually is. Yoga postures teach us how to fully embody the ever-changing flow of life that goes on seemingly without beginning or end. If we see things in this way, then we gain insight into *vinyasa*—the sequences of movements of thought, breath, and mind. In other words, when we practice always and without end, we see that whatever arises in body, heart, and mind—greed, anger, jealousy, laziness, boredom—is recognized as another flowing moment. Patañjali names this *dharma megha samādhi.*

Practically, this means recognizing what is arising from moment to moment in order to become familiar with patterns, much in the same way that we can break down the succession of stills that create the frames of a motion picture. There are patterns that are benign as well as other patterns (of movement, thought, speech, listening) that are so conditioned they stand in the way of immediate experience. The moment you recognize a pattern, you can accept that it is there with patience. Just allow whatever is there to be there. Then keep staying with it. Imagine mind and body like an empty field and whatever pattern you notice it is just moving through; you don't have to identify it as "me" or "mine," but just allow it to live and exist as a pattern. Sometimes this is simply feeling a pattern of a headache or a part of a breath cycle; it might not even be linguistic.

Narratives are only ideas. As persons in bodies, we are like threads made up of multiple strands, each thread being a story about our likes and dislikes. Some strands are continuous over long periods of time, others like the short bits of wool that are spun into yarn; achieve the appearance of continuity only when seen from a sufficient distance. Practice of yoga postures and attention to breath give us the tools to find this distance in order to see the distinction between being in the body and resting in our ideas of the body. The more we let the threads of storytelling dissolve, the closer we come to the experience of life. Then the body becomes something much more reliable. The closer we are to the heartbeat of existence, the less we need the thread of stories. The practice is to move beyond the story line and to stay, with acceptance, patience, and curiosity, with the changing sensations that appear from moment to moment. We move from our idea of "body" to the feeling of an energetic flow of conditions. We become process, and in so doing, come closer to nature. There are some practical ways to do this. This is the practice of *smṛti* (immediate attention). *Smṛti* is best translated as "mindfulness," and mindfulness has several important attributes that deepen as practice matures: present-centered, nonconceptual, nonjudgmental, intentional, engagement through nonattachment, nonverbal, exploratory, liberating, steadiness, and ease.

One practical technique for maintaining focus in each and every movement requires that we keep focused on the body in and of itself, and put aside distraction, attachment, or distress with reference to the world. What this means is recognizing the body as a body, without thinking about it in terms of what it means or what it can do in the world. It could be either good or bad looking. It could be strong or weak. It could be flexible or ill, plagued with cancer or HIV, or robust and energetic. It could be agile or clumsy—all the issues we tend to worry about when we think about the body. Patañjali says, "Put those issues aside; find a sense of the breath, body, mind, and world as indivisible."[2]

Just be with the body in and of itself, sitting right here. When you sit down on your cushion or yoga mat and close your eyes—what do you have? There's the sensation of "bodiness" that you're sitting with. That's your frame of reference. Try to stay with it. Keep bringing the mind back to this sense of the body until it gets the message and begins to settle down. In the beginning of the practice, you find the mind going out to grasp this or that, so you note it enough to tell it to let go, return to the body, and hold on there. Then it goes out to grasp something else, so you tell it to let go, come back, and latch on to the body again. Eventually you reach a point where you can actually grasp hold of the breath and you don't let go. From that point on, whatever else that happens to come into your awareness is like a fish coming up and brushing the back of your hand while you're swimming in a river. At first you note the felt sense of the fish, but once you get used to the fact that there are fish in the water with you, you don't have to continue to notice them. You stay with the body as your basic frame of reference. Other things come and go, you're aware of them, but you don't drop the breath and go running after them. This is when you have really established the body as a solid frame of reference.

That is why we refer to the posture as a label that sets up a frame of reference. Otherwise, we confuse postural-alignment technique for the experience of yoga and continually find ourselves caught as witnesses somehow outside of direct experience.

As you learn to stay present and recirculate energy by being less distracted, you develop some new qualities of mind. One is mindfulness (smṛti). The term *mindfulness* means being able to remember, to keep something in mind. In the *Yoga-Sutra,* sometimes the term *smṛti* is used to connote mindfulness practice and sometimes it refers to the act of remembering. In English we use the term *mindful* in the same way, as a reminder, a way of waking up—"be mindful of your step." A practical way to translate *mindfulness* is as present-centered, nonjudgmental awareness with acceptance. In terms of the body, we could also refer to mindfulness as immediate awareness. In the case of establishing the body as a frame of reference, it means being able to remember where you're supposed to be—with the body—and you don't let yourself forget, whether you are in formal sitting meditation, prāṇāyāma, or āsana.

Another quality that arises though the practices of prāṇāyāma, meditation, and āsana is concentration, which is another means of being aware of what is actually going on in the present. Are you with the body? Are you with the breath? Is the breath comfortable? Simply notice what's actually happening in the present moment. We tend to confuse mindfulness with concentration, but actually they are two separate things: mindfulness means being able to remember where you want to keep your awareness; concentration means that you are absorbed in what you are doing, no longer relating to your action from the place of a separate self. The term *mindfulness* is a term much more familiar to Buddhism than it is to the *Yoga-Sutra,* but nevertheless descriptive of Patañjali's sixth limb, dhāraṇā. Concentration follows naturally from mindfulness. This is why Patañjali describes a movement from āsana (posture) to pratyāhāra (natural uncoupling of sense organs from sense objects) to dhāraṇā (meditation on an object) to dhyāna (absorption) to samādhi (deeper levels of concentration and integration). Don't be put off by terms such as *samādhi* or *concentration* if they are new to you—Patañjali gives very simple and straightforward instructions, not only for how to practice these techniques but why their application is important in working with the habits of mind.

If you realize that the mind has wandered off, you bring it right back. Immediately. You don't let it wander around, sniffing the flowers. Next, when the mind is with its proper frame of reference, we try to be as sensitive as possible to what's going on—not just drifting in the present moment but really trying to penetrate more and more into the subtle details of what's actually happening with the breath or the mind. There is a whole universe even within one breath cycle.

When you practice in this way, you begin to see that these stages or limbs are actually natural outcomes of one another, and you can't help but settle down and get really comfortable with the body in the present moment. That's when you're ready for the next stage in the practice, which is described as being aware of the phenomenon of origination and the phenomenon of passing away. This is a stage where you're trying to understand cause and effect as they happen in the present—in mind and body. Sensations come and go, thoughts come and go; in fact, everything that is perceivable comes and goes. In terms of concentration practice, once you've got the mind to settle down, you want to understand the interaction of cause and effect in the process of concentration so that you can get it to settle down more solidly for longer periods of time in all sorts of situations. To do this, you have to learn about how things arise and pass away in the mind and body, not by simply watching them but by actually getting involved in their arising and passing away. Staying with the breath means studying it as it arises and also as it passes away, feeling sensations as they arise and disband.

The link and successive progression from limb to limb is important to understand, especially once the first four limbs have been established. Once attention internalizes and the body is fit for being still, we focus the mind on an object. Most meditation practices begin as concentration practices, because one is honing in on a particular field of focus. So a characteristic of the last three limbs—dhāraṇā, dhyāna, and samādhi—is that each begins with concentration exercises using appropriate objects on which one focuses. In this procedure, however, once a certain level of concentration is achieved so that undistracted focusing can be maintained, one goes on to examine, with steady, careful attention and in great detail, all sensory and mental processes. Through this contemplation, we learn how to notice all experience from a place of stillness.

Meditation practice is best pursued under the guidance of a teacher.

The mind has such a strong pull toward identifying with the contents of experience or thinking "I've got it" that it's helpful to have someone to guide you through the nooks and crannies of meditation, even if only to offer encouragement when practice is difficult. The aim is to achieve total and immediate awareness, or mindfulness, of all phenomena. This leads eventually to the full and clear perception of the impermanence of all phenomena and the complete separation of awareness from all that is perceived. This separation is paradoxically undivided and free of subject and object. Patañjali calls it *kaivalya.* While *kaivalya* is often translated as referring to the aloofness or isolation of the yogi, it is rather the distinct difference between *puruṣa,* meaning "pure awareness," and *prakṛti,* which refers to all changing phenomena.

Patañjali doesn't make it clear if the path of dhāraṇā, or meditation on an object, can lead to kaivalya or even freedom from duḥkha. It seems that one has to move on toward deeper states of absorption matched with a thorough grounding in ethical conduct in order to move into sustained modes of pure awareness. While the former leads to temporarily altered states of consciousness, it is the latter that leads to enduring and thoroughgoing changes in the person and paves the way to achieving wholeness.

Psychologically, the practical implications of meditation are quite clear. The meditative experiences, when properly carried out and developed, lead to greater ability to concentrate, greater freedom from distraction, greater tolerance of change and turmoil around and inside oneself, and sharper awareness and greater alertness about one's own responses, both physical and mental. They also lead, more generally, to greater calmness or tranquillity. Through meditation practice, coupled with strong ethical practices, we learn to develop a wisdom that acts as an antidote to the predispositions, imprints, ongoing habits, and deluded states of mind that so often dominate our day-to-day existence. This kind of letting go allows us to be completely open in all of our relationships and helps us act wisely and without self-interest in any given situation.

Spiritual experience is never a complete, unmediated, spontaneous expression as long as the subtlest kind of conceptual distinction is present. This takes us to one of the simplest aspects of practice: being honest. Once we train the mind to see the body as the body, to be with the breath without distraction, and to stay present even during difficult mental and physical states, a natural outcome is being honest about what we see. Sometimes the way we perceive our own experience is so wrapped up in preference and self-image that we don't even know what our own body looks and feels like independent of our ideas of ourselves. Definitions of self are mostly sluggish and eternally escape any accurate measurement or likeness. "The world is like an experience that has no witness," we are told in the *Yoga Vāsiṣṭa.*[3] What constitutes reality in any given moment is inseparable from our perception.

The psychological benefit of getting to know the body, breath, and mind without conceptual proliferation is learning how to see honestly, without attachment or aversion. From here, being truthful in other relationships is relatively easy, and suddenly we are cultivating the yama of satya, or truthfulness and honesty. Otherwise, the *nadi*s remain clogged with self-image, and self-image is based on raga (attachment) and dveṣa (aversion) and a never-ending, solipsistic story self-generated by the ahaṇkāra. One story in the *Yoga Vāsiṣṭa* describes a man whose stories of self, like insubstantial clouds, are mistaken for truth.

> There was once a man made by a magic machine [Mayayantramaya], a stupid idiot. He lived all by himself in an empty place, like a mirage in a desert. Everything else was just a reflection of him, but the fool didn't realize this. As he got old, he thought, The sky is mine and I will rule over it, and so he made a house out of air in the sky in order to rule over the air and the sky. But after a while the house faded away. He cried out, "Oh, my house made of space, where have you gone?" And he built another, and another, and another, and

> all of them dispersed into the air, and he went on lamenting for them.[4]

Commenting on this parable, the *Yoga Vāsiṣṭa* says that the man represents the egoity of the "I"-maker (ahaṇkāra) and the houses are the various manifestations of the body, or physical existence. The man does not realize that his creations are all mental constructions. The "I"-maker will always pump out fantasies, but the key is allowing them to have free play without identification or reification. Even fantasies of what the soul is, what it is made of, and where it comes from, are all activities of a mind wanting to create security. One of the key mechanisms of the ahaṇkāra, once it realizes the limits of material existence, is to create a metaphysical existence. This metaphysical existence, usually in the form of stories that make sense of one's place in the world, become problematic when taken to be literal truths. But what is most problematic is the literalization of an essential self whose essence we think we can know. The union inherent in the basic axiomatic definition of the term *yoga* is not metaphysical speculation about our inherent soul but rather a raw experience of the contingent nature of our present conditions and the freedom that arrives with such insight. The breath, body, and mind belong to no one, nor are they completely independent. Yoga teaches us to live comfortably in contradictions without having to resolve them, because beneath the layers and layers of conceptual designations imputed to things via the mind, all opposites are inherently resolved; everything begins without separation.

# 17. *Prāṇa* and *Citta*

THE UNION OF BODY and mind or self and soul, or whatever way the modern split is described, is first healed with breath. We are a culture that does not breathe. There is no life without prāṇa, and there is no death without life. The world turns on the cycle of the breath, not just in human form but across the entire living spectrum. Again, prāṇa is not just breathing per se, but the life force that animates existence. What does not breathe or move this vital energy efficiently dies quickly. The breath, in yoga, returns us to the present and always acts as the path itself if there is any internal movement to consider. We turn inward most easily by focusing on the breath.

If we are privileged to be present at either the birth or the death of another human being, we can watch them come into the world inhaling or depart exhaling. From the first autonomous breath, we pass this life energy back and forth between us. The mother passes on physical existence to the child by means of the breath. Breathing is devotion to life.

Prāṇa (breathing, life energy) and citta (consciousness, mind) are two aspects of the same energetic cycle. In *The Tree of Yoga*, B.K.S. Iyengar writes,

> The *Hatha Yoga Pradīpika* says that yoga is prāṇa-vṛtti-nirodha —stilling the fluctuations of the breath. Patañjali's *Yoga-Sutras* say that yoga is chitta-vṛtti-nirdodha—stilling the fluctuations of the mind. The mind can go in many directions

> in a split second. Its movements are very fast and varied. But the breath cannot go in many directions at once. It has only one path: inhalation and exhalation. It can pause for a moment in a state of retention, but it cannot multiply like the mind. According to the *Hatha Yoga Pradīpika,* controlling the breath and observing its rhythm brings the consciousness to stillness. Thus, though the *Hatha Yoga Pradīpika* begins with the control of prāṇa, breath or energy, and Patañjali's *Yoga-Sutras* begin with the control of consciousness, yet they meet at a certain point where there is no difference between them. By controlling the breath you are controlling consciousness, and by controlling consciousness you bring rhythm to the breath.[1]

When we pay attention to the breath, we watch its flow through the prism of the body, and one of the helpful ways of feeling the route of the breath is by understanding the role of the nadis. The nadis route the energy of the breath and can be likened to the bank of a river or the walls of a tunnel. Traditionally, Hatha Yoga was the domain of Tantra Yoga. The language of Hatha Yoga is a language that describes patterns of energy and the means of stilling and sculpting those patterns. Hatha Yoga is the detailed investigation of the breath, mind, and body through feeling, visualization, chanting, and direct observation—all of which are techniques that one refines until the internal body becomes still and centered. Much like stilling the fluctuations of the mind, the Hatha Yoga or Tantric practitioner uses the immediate sensations in the body and breath as a doorway into the nature and functioning of the mind. This is very practical: when we breathe, there is a flow of energy, called prāṇa, which moves through the body and mind. What does prāṇa flow through? All thought and movement float on this current of prāṇa, and prāṇa flows through the nadis. Look into the pathways of the nadis and it's hard not to marvel at the microcosm of life manifest in the body in the form of fluctuating sensations, pulsations, minuscule worlds inside minuscule worlds.

The nadis are like nerves, vessels, meridians, or ducts through which prāṇa flows in mind and body. The nadis transport prāṇa through the body and mind and interestingly do not end at the perimeter of the body but extend out into the world beyond the body. Through visualization and prāṇāyāma technique, one follows prāṇa through the conduits of the nadis. It is easy to follow the breath through immediate feeling as well as visualization so that we notice and feel where it moves in the body; the route of its movement becomes the starting point for the meditation. Meditating on the energetic flow of the breath and visualizing the nadis brings mind, breath, and body together in a seamless unity of attention. Without identifying with personal thoughts or feelings, when the mind is concentrated in the flow of the breath, especially through the simple act of feeling, we experience a radical departure from our normal mode of perceiving the body, the world, and ourselves. When the mind is focused on one particular thing, in this case the energetic flow and weave of the breath, our focus becomes so microscopic that the mind becomes quite clear and effortlessly radiant. Experience now comes and goes with ease because mind and breath, mediated by a calm and unconditioned nervous system, become very still and receptive; the breath moves quietly, as does the mind, but there is no reactivity or lack, like the quiet blooming of an iris or the silken threads of light.

In the *Yoga Vāsiṣṭa,* Vāsiṣṭa tells Rama,

> "The prāṇa is indistinguishably united with the mind. In fact, the consciousness that tends toward thinking, on account of the movement of prāṇa, is known as the mind. Movement of thought in the mind arises from movement of prāṇa; and movement of prāṇa arises because of movement of thought in consciousness. They form a cycle of mutual dependence, like waves and movements of currents in water."[2]

One cannot speak of vinyasa, or movements of the mind-body without also describing the movement of breath, as they are essentially interdependent. Most people associate vinyasa with the movement of linking postures together; however, there are other ways of understanding it. *Vinyasa* also refers to the movements of thought (*citta vṛtti*), movements within a breath cycle (*prāṇa vāyuu*), and cyclical movement within the circulatory, respiratory, and immune systems.

We all know that some steadiness of breathing brings about steadiness in the mind-body. Vāsiṣṭa continues,

> . . . the mind is caused by the movements of prāṇa; and hence by the stilling of prāṇa; the mind becomes still. . . . The movement of mind and prāṇa becomes still when desire (in the form of clinging) comes to an end in one's own heart. . . . [T]he movement of prāṇa is also stilled by the effortless practice of breathing, without strain. This also occurs when you bring the end of an exhale (as retention) to a standstill for longer and longer periods of time.[3]

Vāsiṣṭa instructs Rama in breathing practice in order to demonstrate how perception of the world is continually influenced by one's state of mind and body. Stilling the tendency toward clinging, conceptualizing, and reacting to the world comes about through correct breathing. Breathing without effort is the key to stilling the mind. Stilling the mind allows the habits of thought to recede and the world to appear immediately, without the obstacles of concepts getting in the way of direct experience. First we stretch the breath and press it through the nadi tubes, especially where certain knots exist, then once the breath is exercised, we leave it alone and feel its unmodified rhythm.

The knots in the nadis are symptoms of larger holding patterns that we call "the saṁskāras." The saṁskāras are undone when one creates the conditions for a steady and uninterrupted flow of prāṇa through the nadis. It is most helpful to think of the saṁskāras as structural holding patterns that influence the feeling pathways called "nadis." Steady flow occurs when prāṇa (breath, energy) and citta (mind, consciousness) come together and move as one. When the breath and mind move together as one, the central channels of the body open to the present moment, which is none other than what is occurring now. Like tracing a sound back to its source or seeing the water that makes up a wave, we keep the mind so intimately connected to the breath that the two become inseparable. In yoga we follow everything to the vanishing edge, where form becomes absence, and what appears as empty is brought forward again into the world of form. This is why we practice yoga postures as a form of prāṇāyāma, which in turn is a practice of meditation.

When we move toward integrating āsana practice and prāṇāyāma, postural alignment serves the respiratory system, and all alignment techniques become rituals of devotion in service of inhaling and exhaling. Because the mind has to focus on a movement without distraction in order to follow the breath, āsana as a form of prāṇāyāma, interiorizes awareness (*pratyāhāra*) and sets the mind and body in concentration (dhyāna).

Exploring yoga postures psychologically, physically, and energetically allows us to access depths of yoga practice, where many different paths come together. T.K.V. Desikachar describes the tendency to see the various approaches in yoga as leading to separate goals as superficial: "Primarily it is a question of our state of mind. Whatever happens in the mind and causes a change in it affects the whole person, including the body and all experiences on a physical level."[4]

Mind and body operate in unity, as do the various limbs and methods of yoga. Desikachar continues:

> People often ask me if I teach āsanas, and when I answer "Yes," they say: "Oh, then you are a hatha yogi!" If I am talking about the *Yoga-Sutra* they say "Oh, you are a rāja yogi!" If I say that I recite the Vedas the comment is: "Oh, so you are a mantra

> yogi!" If I simply say that I practice yoga, they do not know what to make of me. Many people want to give everything and everyone a label. Unfortunately, these classifications have become much too important and give the impression that there are fundamental differences between the various forms of yoga. But really they are all dealing with the same thing, and are only looking at them from different perspectives. If we really follow one direction in yoga as far as we can go, then it will lead us along all paths of yoga.[5]

Unless the limb of āsana practice is not explored to its depth—meaning looking into the actions not just of body but also of mind, breath, and energetic flow—we won't penetrate fully the yoga of āsana. Don't be caught in the superficial geometry of yoga postures without tending to and tuning in to the quality of the gaze, the spreading of the breath, the pauses at the end and beginning of every breath cycle, and the diaphragmatic action of the *bandha*s, as these internal forms of alignment draw the mind into concentration and insight, without which the mind remains at the periphery of yoga āsana.

## *Flow and Stability*

In Tantric terms, we can call the process of prāṇa "energy flow." Fluctuating patterns of energy in the body, like fluctuations in the mind, become steady through correct breathing and immediate attention, and the interesting thing is that good technique requires the attention that we are trying to cultivate in all the other limbs. All techniques, when not turned into doctrine, become mindfulness practices—they give the mind a specific place to focus so that we can drop into levels of absorption that interrupt distraction and habit. When the mind enters into any action fully, when we are completely present to what is unfolding as it unfolds, the fluctuations of citta settle into nirodha.

When energy can flow through the body uninterrupted by latent physical or psychological tendencies, consciousness settles and the equilibrium of the kośas is reached. This is not esoteric but simply practical psychophysiology based on verifiable experience in the here and now. When mind and breath settle into each other, the nervous system responds and the body unconditions itself. Like a rock that is heavy, water that is wet, a sky that is open and endless, the body too has its equilibrium, its essential way of being as it is. When prāṇa and citta flow together, the saṁskāras in the mind-body begin to dissolve, because the attributes that give rise to the saṁskāras dissolve when there is no clinging or constriction in either mind or body.

There is no posture without energy flow. In fact, any living organism depends on energy flow. However, the process does not stop there. The flow of prāṇa is not sufficient in and of itself; it is energy storage, and capturing that is key. For example, the sun shines on Earth and it also gives light to Mars and Venus, but only Earth has life, as far as we know, because only Earth can successfully capture and store sunlight. The action that enables life to occur is really the way in which an energy circle can be closed. When energy is flowing in a circle, we have a life cycle as it were, which stores and feeds on the energy flow within those specific conditions. Something magical happens within a circle, a maṇḍala. A circle means perpetual return, and perpetual return gives stability. This is what we call "dynamic stability."

A yoga posture is a perfect model of dynamic stability. When we close an energy circle, through focused attention, correct breathing, and the application of bandhas, the prāṇa in the body and mind begins to flow through new channels and also unclogs previously knotted channels. This unknotting only occurs, however, when prāṇa is coherent, steady, and recirculating. The nadis are like meridians through which prāṇa flows. But sometimes prāṇa cannot flow clearly because the tubes through which the energy of the breath flows are clogged up.

Notice, for instance, how when you inhale and exhale there are parts of that cycle that are smooth and places where the breath ripples or skips or feels constricted. It is usually when the prāṇa flow is interrupted at these sites of physical holding that the mind gets distracted. Prāṇa and citta move together; they are two sides of the same coin. Even if you listen to the sound of the breath, you will notice that sometimes the breath sounds smooth and sometimes it is interrupted by little fluctuations. When the breath fluctuates, so does the mind.

Swami Rama describes the way these winds of the breath effect the functioning of the entire mind-body process:

> Breath is an external manifestation of the force of prāṇa. Breath is the fly-wheel that regulates the entire machine of the body. Just as the control of the fly-wheel of an engine controls all the other mechanisms in it, so the control of the external breath leads to control of the gross and subtle, physical and mental aspects of our life machine.[6]

The Tantric model of prāṇa expresses physiologically what the *Yoga-Sutra* describes psychologically. It is said that there are 72,000 nadis in the body; together they form an extremely fine network of subtle channels spread throughout the ethereal body (body of prāṇa, pranic sheath, or energetic body). Most disease or inflexibility is the result of congestion, blocks, or restrictions in the nadi system. The nadis are psychological as well, so when you talk of psychological hindrances, anxieties, neurotic tendencies, or obstacles, we also use the language of the nadis. Psychological knots exist within the nadis in the same way that overturned logs or beaver dams interrupt the smooth flow of a river. The breath always wants to flow uninterrupted, and the interruptions in the cycles of the breath, known by means of distraction or agitation in mind and body, becomes the place where we focus our attention and also reveals the next step on the path. All symptoms act this way—as signals for our attention and as road markers on the path.

The importance of the *iḍā, piṅgalā,* and *suṣumnā* nadis is well developed in Tantric texts and also forms the basis of Pattabhi Jois's teachings of āsana and prāṇāyāma. Pattabhi Jois teaches correct breathing, gazing, and bandhas in order to achieve good pranic flow through the nadis. B.K.S. Iyengar uses the same terminology. Kṛṣṇamacharya, when he went to Tibet to study yoga, returned to the practice of Hatha Yoga, subtle attention to the energetic elements of practice. When yoga posture sequences are practiced from the inside out, meaning that the mind is with not just the physical movement but the subtle movements of breath and energy, attention interiorizes and the posture practice becomes a Tantric one.

> To preserve energies in the body and prevent their dissipation, āsanas and mudras (seals), prāṇāyāmas and bandhas . . . were prescribed. The heat so generated causes the kuṇḍalinī to uncoil. The serpent lifts its head, enters the suṣumnā and is forced up through the chakras one by one to the sahasrāra.[7]

This passage by B.K.S. Iyengar describes how attention and breath flow through the meridians of the body until the energy in the pelvic floor, in the form of kuṇḍalinī, begins to move through the channels, especially the central axis of the body (suṣumnā). Later in his description of kuṇḍalinī in *Light on Yoga,* B.K.S. Iyengar describes the serpent as an "allegory" that denotes the movement of vital energy.[8] What is important here is the way that kuṇḍalinī represents in image form the clear movement of energy within the meridians of the body. The energy can only move through the body when attention is present. As we press the breath through the nadis, we are also stretching the mind through the nadis. And kuṇḍalinī is representative of a mind that moves with the breath as one as they course through the nervous system and dissolve the distractions and mental toxins that previously obstructed the clear passage of energy through the systems of the body.

Kuṇḍalinī is not the breath itself but rather the energetic aspect of the life force manifested only in part as the breath. It's helpful to return to the etymological significance of the word *kuṇḍalinī,* from the verb *kuṇda,* meaning "to burn." Kuṇḍalinī is the burning up of knots and holding patterns in mind and body, the most significant of which is the clinging to self-image. This may explain why many people describe "kuṇḍalinī rising" as both full of physical sensation and also mental fear. Abiniveśa, the fear of letting go of self-image, is always at work in any process of letting go.

Hatha Yoga and Tantra Yoga are inseparable when practiced from the inside out, because the essence of Hatha Yoga has always been Tantra. In fact, what took the great teacher Kṛṣṇamacharya out of India and into Tibet was his search for someone to put the Tantra back into the physical postures of Hatha Yoga. He needed someone to help him find the subtle energetics or psychological dimensions of the physical practice of yoga.

Prāṇa flows where citta goes. Thus, we steady the eyes so that attention and the breath, citta and prāṇa, come together. Bandhas are conjunctions of energy that act as valves to recirculate energy within the nadis so that prāṇa does not leak from the body. Practicing breathing, gazing, and bandhas simultaneously creates a closed loop of energetic flow within the nadis. This is called "pratyāhāra," which refers to the natural uncoupling of sense organs from sense objects when the breath and attention flow as one. When energy increases in the body during posture and breathing practices, it always attempts to reorganize the internal energetic systems of the mind-body. When the pressure is turned up, the system begins to change if the energy can recirculate. If the energy dissipates, the flow increases but conditioning of the system remains unchanged. Unless we can allow this to happen naturally by setting up the condition for good energy flow, the flow will temporarily increase and then become fragmented. In breathing practices, we pay very close attention to the eyes so that as new and more challenging energetic waves move through the body, there is no distraction. Distraction is always common in the eyes, because we are so used to having hungry eyes, always looking externally. This does not mean being stiff trying to be perfectly steady but setting up the intention to face and host whatever occurs in immediate awareness.

The iḍā, on the right side of the body, descending from the bridge of the right nasal passage, is generally associated with the moon, white in color, and with the prāṇa or rising vital breath and Śiva (male energy); the piṅgalā on the left side of the body, descending from the left nasal passage, with the sun, the color red, blood, the descending apānic breath and Śākti (female energy).

The central channel, or suṣumnā, is associated with fire and the union of the iḍā, and piṅgalā. Pattabhi Jois calls the suṣumnā nadi, which runs from the center of the pelvic floor through to the crown of the head, "the empty flute." The term *kuṇḍalinī,* which has been fetishized and imbued with literalist interpretations (such as a purely physical feeling of tingling up the spine), reduces the essence of that process. "Kuṇḍalinī" describes in metaphorical language the present moment that is curled up but inaccessible in every movement of experience in which there is even an ounce of self-image. We are not present because of karmic patterns, most notably greed, hatred, and delusion.

The work of correct breathing, attention, gazing, and alignment within any yoga posture is aimed at smoothing out the fluctuating patterns of citta and prāṇa within the nadis and among the different sheaths of the body, by the act of being present even in times of distraction. Even when caught in turbulent thoughts or emotions, we return to the breath and, in doing so, calm the fluctuations in mind and nervous system. Over time, the calmness becomes easier to find, and you can establish the calmness as the basis for further practice. Kuṇḍalinī is a metaphor for present experience free of the scaffolding created by the mind's preferences. When the nadis open and kuṇḍalinī uncoils and flows through the suṣumnā, we can understand this as the removal of any psychophysical bias that interrupts the opportunity to be present. Like a serpent representing the profundity of now, kuṇḍalinī speaks of nothing beyond itself. Like the present moment, it is present by its absence and thus requires of the practitioner focus and relaxed attention to what is currently and constantly occurring within the body during a single breath cycle. Kuṇḍalinī is aroused as the present movement is appreciated—not through conception but through the simple act of breathing itself. It's the breath that wakes the serpent, like a rock ledge that sets up the fall of water.

In breathing practices, including yoga postures, we are looking for a clean, uninterrupted flow of energy, which sets up the ideal maṇḍala, or energy cycle. Every maṇḍala, or every cycle of energy, is a home of stored coherent energy. Coherent energy comes together and moves within channels of a cycle so that it can do its work gracefully, as opposed to incoherent energy, which goes in all directions and remains distracted and unstable. Incoherent energy is prāṇa that moves through overly conditioned channels of thought, feeling, perception, sensation, and movement. We are looking for clean, uninterrupted flow.

If there is past injury or strong places of holding, the energy flow is decreased, interrupted, or rerouted. Sometimes holding patterns are reversed and instead of resistance there is a lack of resistance. For example, if there is a place without any resistance, such as a misplaced hip or an overfunctioning nervous system, or even a personality with weak boundaries, the prāṇa flows too much.

The interesting thing here is that the tendency of prāṇa is to flow with a balanced velocity, with an intuited smoothness. A smooth flow of prāṇa creates graceful movement, a calm nervous system, and a steady mind. The energy in the body is always aiming to improve circulation and steadiness of flow, much like the flow of a river. DNA is constantly being altered, cells are always letting go of previous patterns of control, and tissues are always working to rid themselves of the chemicals that we ingest. A major key in persevering our continuity is the ability of body's systems to right countless small wrongs that bombard the body and mind at every instant. We adapt; we change our molecular responses, we repair ourselves, all in the service of keeping the gyroscope of the mind-body spinning smoothly. It is this constant flux that enables dynamic stability and the motion of stillness. Even what we think of as constant—bones, self, movement—is constantly changing in order to maintain the dynamic equilibrium of cellular life that allows the dynamic equilibrium of our lives in the world. The changing constancy of living beings underlies the homeostasis of our ecological existence and demonstrates firsthand the teaching that everything that is perceivable (prakṛti) is provisional and contingent.

Our minds and bodies are always limited by their origins. Change in mind and body means being stretched out of what is known in order to sow the seeds of openness to what is unknown, and that is why change and transformation is more a matter of loss than it is of growth. The language of growth tends to become personal, entrepreneurial, and ambitious. Taking on the new is always easier than letting go of what is old, because what is historical is what is known and comfortable. Sometimes we are so used to, so caught up in, our ways of moving and being that we don't see them as stale or outmoded until symptoms appear to tell us so. The first step in working with our conditioned minds and bodies is seeing what is old in the first place. Then we can let it go. We have a home in the present moment whenever we arrive.

# 18. The Empty Vessel

The root of "spirit" is the Latin *spirare,* to breathe. Whatever lives on the breath, then, must have its spiritual dimension.

—Jane Hirshfield

There is no body to speak of, just a flow of conditions, empty of an inherent identity; a yoga posture allows us to experience this energetically. But it requires focus and patience and the ability to see clearly and stay with the difficult moments that arise when the prāṇa meets deep holding patterns and we want to get away, become distracted, or be anywhere other than here. There is no way to escape. The fear of letting go into the reality of what is, is nothing other than giving up a fixed self-image; this kind of fear is the self running away from its inherent intimacy with all things, vast, unknowable, always changing. Li Po writes,

The birds have vanished down the sky.
Now the last cloud drains away.

We sit together, the mountain and me,
until only the mountain remains.[1]

A yoga posture is not a self-enclosed static entity but an organic cycle—an open movement. The body and mind come alive when the senses converge in the world. It is through the engagement with what is not "me" that I participate in the world via body and mind. When mind and body are flexible and the sense organs less polluted, kuṇḍalinī, in the form of prāṇa, begins to flow uninterruptedly.

When we are fully in an action, the technique brings us to a point, like crossing a river in a raft, where we no longer need the technique; once we have crossed, we no longer need the vehicle. First the technique drops and then the conceptualizations drop and then feeling like a self falls away until there is movement and perception and sensation but one is so fully in the movement that there is nobody there. There is movement with no mover. There is a yoga pose, but there is nobody practicing. Like never-ending sky over endless mountains, being who you are in the most elegant sense tolerates even discursive thoughts and strong emotions but rejects nothing.

Pleasure and pain are such a major part of our perceptual lives. It's almost a strange occurence in nature to be so focused on these two realms. Through the practice of yoga postures, we learn to move deeply within postures from the inside out so that our kinesthetic experience is dominant, not our modes of preference. We feel something so internally that we simply dissolve into movement and feeling, even with activity in the mind, but there is no sign of an agent. Then the internal dimension of yoga opens up.

This is the mystical side of yoga, which is nothing more than deep experience of the present conditions. If we cling to any of these wonderful moments, then the yoga practice returns us to the superficial level of a "me" that needs to "have" an experience. When we have profound experiences in yoga, such as direct contact with strong energies or clear insights, we have to also be vigilant that the mind does not overinterpret those experiences as special. It is easy to give such experiences authority, but this would also be a form of ego-clinging. Whether rare or regular, when energy moves, states of mind surface. If one could abide permanently in such deep states of being, it would imply great skill concentrating, but this is not liberation. Samādhi is not the goal of yoga.

In the last chapter of the *Yoga-Sutra,* Patañjali states that deep meditative concentration is a skill but not the goal, because there can still be clinging even to those states. What these states do offer, however, is a state of mind, body, and heart that is free from the strong pull of materialism, and this is most valuable in a mind, body, and culture that always have dangling the potential for grasping and reward.

Yoga postures have always been considered a Tantric practice, because working with the physical body brings you into direct contact with energy flow, the nervous system, the breath, and the visualizing mind. A yoga posture is an invitation into the kinesthetic sense of being everything and at the same time being nothing. It is the awakening from the illusion of a separate me, a separate body, and the feeling of fragmentation. We have talked about this from the perspective of mind and body. Nondual practice is the thread that weaves together sutra (psychological study) and Tantra (energetic movement in mind and body) to achieve the same goal: keeping mind and body alert and open to their own transformation.

We are not so different from trees and water and birds. We are of course humans and not other species, so we must ask, what does it mean to be essentially human? What occurs psychologically when we are finally free to be lost in the world without self-reference, without needing to treat our experiences in terms of a separate "me"? What does it mean to leave the other, be it person or world, untreated? This occurs not just by knowledge but through practice and connection, theory and engagement, so that one flows from the self across the magical bridge of sensitivity that leads out into the world and back again. What happens when we become the mirror behind us rather than checking ourselves endlessly in the mirror in front of us? What is it that obscures our basic nature?

What obstructs our basic nature, what Pattabhi Jois calls "the enemies in the heart," is our habitual clinging to duality. This clinging is reinforced over and again, because it takes a fair amount of stillness and reflection to notice how the way that we experience life is limited by the conditioned grooves we call the saṁskāras. That is why yoga postures and meditation are so important—they show us how limiting these grooves are. Yoga postures train us to be free of clinging to duality. This begins by bringing together and essentially fusing the breath and the mind. When the mind and breath are brought together in an action, duality dissolves, disappears, vanishes! What remains is boundless and outside of time; Patañjali calls this *śūnyatā* (emptiness). Or it is called the *paramātman* (the selfless self of awareness). Patañjali also calls the experience of nonduality the *puruṣa,* which is empty of self-form (*svarūpa śūnya*). Patañjali gives this pure awareness a name, "puruṣa," but the name itself is, of course, not "puruṣa."

Where does winter get its snow? Where does spring arrive from? The Buddhists are always challenging the Hindus on whether there is a true self (*ātman*) or nothing one can call self (*anātman*). Patañjali stakes the middle ground between these two systems, and in doing so he creates a paradox that many traditions have tried to resolve through convenient interpretation. For example, when one looks through the innumerable English translation of the *Yoga-Sutra,* almost no one translates the word *śūnyatā.* But when we look into what the Indian tradition calls "self," it is the selfless self that is no self at all! Here is an excerpt from a lecture Robert Thurman gave at a yoga studio in Manhattan:

> Student: Isn't the traditional Indian teaching of the self in direct opposition to the Buddhist teaching of emptiness?
>
> Thurman: That is superficial. Opposing those systems in that way makes no inroads into what they are actually about. What is the self?
>
> Student: Well, it's the opposite of emptiness.

> Thurman: No, no, no, the Indians would say. *Neti, neti* (it's not that, it's not that). The self is not your body, not your eye, not your mind, not your thoughts, not your perception, it's not you or any "thing" for that matter. No, no, no.[2]

All traditions use words to answer and describe, with varied effectiveness, this experience of stillness and oneness with the nature of things. Puruṣa is a way of being without becoming, like being a form of life rather than a somebody.

In this book I have focused on the way śūnyatā has been used by Patañjali to point out a paradox, namely that from the point of view of the practitioner, pure awareness (śūnyatā) is the felt experience of nonduality (samādhi). However, as soon as we use words, we find ourselves caught up in dualistic language. Great Buddhist teachers such as Nāgārjuna, and especially those in the Mahayana traditions, have been able to turn language inside out and on its head until we no longer get stuck using concepts to describe the meditative state of complete integration. Patañjali gives the state a name—puruṣa—and in so doing creates a paradox that scholars have argued about ever since. Yet from the perspective of the yoga practitioner, the experience of samādhi is identical to the Buddhist notion of śūnyatā, and Patañjali uses both terms in the *Yoga-Sutra* and creates a kind of artificial fence upon which he rests. He does not think puruṣa is an entity, as the dualistic tradition of Sāṅkhya Yoga claims, and he does not deconstruct the language used to describe puruṣa in the way the Buddha might have. Nevertheless, from the internal perspective of the yogi, he is describing the same experience. Perhaps the term *puruṣa* is the only thing that keeps the *Yoga-Sutra* from becoming a Buddhist text!

To be liberated is to be free from clinging, even to concepts. When we begin yoga posture practice, it feels as though there is a solid "me" practicing with this solid body. But over time, the sense of "I" shifts, and we notice that. The body is pliable and not static, and we notice that too. In fact the "I" is not dependent on the body, and the body is not dependent on the "I." Yoga postures allow us to dismantle our fixation on the permanence of what we experience. We usually cling to the content of our experience as being that—not just as something that is being experienced but as something with solidity that is real, solid, permanent. But when we look honestly, especially from a place of stillness, we see that experience is simply experience, and it is not made of anything solid whatsoever. Experience is simply an empty cognition.

When the saṁskāras are seen for what they are—conditioned patterns or potentials that influence clinging and misapprehension—then they can be seen through. This is what is meant by *śūnyatā* (emptiness). When we are with experience as experience, the heart opens and is bottomless; when the subject disappears, so does the object and vice versa. This is simply one heart, one mind, immediate awareness. The heart opens when there is no clinging in mind and body.

One of the most famous passages from the Upaniṣads, in which Yājñavalka speaks to his wife, Maitreyi, describes the way in which the nature of a moment, when seen for what it is, reveals the boundlessness of reality. Notice the paradoxical language and Yājñavalka (or the author's) way of pushing past definitions: "Arising out of the elements (*bhūta*), into them also one vanishes away. After death there is no consciousness (*ne pretya samjna sti*)."[3]

Shocked by this, Maitreyi asks him to continue:

> "For where there is a duality, as it were, there one sees another. . . . But when, verily, everything has become just one's own self, then what could one see and through what? . . . Through what could one know that owing to which all this is known? So, through what could one understand the understander? This Self. . . . is imperceptible, for it is never perceived."[4]

How can we name something "self" if it is impossible to perceive, and is therefore no "thing" at all? What Yājñavalka is saying here is that when one realizes nonduality, dualistic consciousness dissolves. When the self dissolves, so too does the object. "Self" in this case refers to the boundlessness of reality, the empty nature of things as they are.

In the Abrahamic religions of Judaism, Christianity, and Islam, in very broad terms, the human person is seen as needing repentance, divine forgiveness, and renewal. The Absolute, for these allied traditions, is an omnipotent, anthropomorphically envisioned, monotheistic godhead. In Buddhism, it is taught that the human person is experiencing suffering unnecessarily due to mistakenly perceiving himself or herself as an enduring, self-conscious entity. Liberation, in Buddhism, begins with the realization that there is no eternal self, but only momentary states that give the illusion of a permanent person. The final extinction of the human person in the form of nirvāna (literally "blowing out") is thus the goal. This is quite similar to Patañjali's description of nirodha. The Absolute, in Buddhist terms, is correlated with śūnya, boundlessness, emptiness. For Buddhism, there is no god per se, nor any other permanent metaphysical reality. For Hinduism, the human existential dilemma is caused by ignorance (avidyā) of our true state as permanent spiritual beings (ātman), and our illusion (maya) of separation from reality. Liberation (mokṣa) is achieved by transcending this illusion, and by realizing our inherent union (yoga) with reality. Speaking in the most general of terms, the absolute reality in Hinduism, and more specifically in Advaita Vedanta (*advaita* literally means "not two") is termed "Brahman" even though Brahman is non-anthropormorphic, and certainly not a "thing."

Each of these traditions holds a very different account of what constitutes our true spiritual nature; each has its own distinctive idea of what it means to realize our true nature; and each has a uniquely divergent idea of what is the ultimate nature of the Absolute. Yoga seems to move within all of these traditions quite comfortably since Patañjali, as an example, and also texts such as the *Yoga Vāsiṣṭa* and *Hatha Yoga Pradīpika,* use language purposely borrowed from other traditions in a way that asks the practitioner to move beyond the doctrine of systems in order to see what those systems are pointing toward. The yogi does not look toward her practices as metaphors of consolation, and in this sense we could call Patañjali's approach toward reality an agnostic one. Standing on the threshold of imagination but firmly planted in present experience, the yogi is concerned with freeing the mind and responding to present circumstances without self-created entrapments. In an increasingly interconnected world, we come to see that yoga is everywhere and everything and that the human being is compassion.

I have chosen these three broad religious traditions (Abrahamic, Buddhist, Hindu) to illustrate the point that not only are there different religions but there are also different categorical types of religion. The point is that these may not be different systems talking about the same thing but rather different systems talking about different types of experience. What is so fascinating (and also difficult) about yoga is that it slides between these different traditions by pointing out the limits of having a system in the first place. Patañjali talks about emptiness and also about puruṣa, pure awareness, creating a paradox of sorts but also appealing to those who have no problem being in between systems. He teaches on the emptiness of self-form (svarūpa śūnya) and also on the tool of using a personal deity (*īśvara-praṇidhānā*) for meditation practice.

The shadow side of this is that there is no network of yoga temples or priests that determine who is and who isn't practicing, who can and who can't be a teacher. The benefit of such a nondualist, agnostic, and anarchic reading of this tradition is that many practitioners have to go deep into texts and practices in order to embody and realize the basic teachings of yoga, free from the constraint of overly rigid doctrine. The shadow of such a viewpoint is that since there is no systematized approach to teaching, and many people simply turn yoga into whatever they want, leading to a self-styled practice that does not avoid the ego's tricks and games. Of course we are going to interpret tradition—that is how it comes alive in each and every one of us and becomes a dynamic cultural process rather than something imagined as timeless and developed in a cultural vacuum. Attending a yoga class at any popular studio is a fascinating and disconcerting study of the way in which people sculpt yoga into whatever they would like it to be. Many teachers use their certification as a modern "yoga teacher" to simply articulate their personal philosophy on life, sometimes without ever having had a teacher of their own. Yoga is a complex and intimate set of interrelated practices that inform every aspect of life, creating a coherent path toward liberation by understanding the causes of suffering and the path to freedom. Hopefully some of the ideas in this book will help practitioners in their approach to practice so that we can all be affected by yoga theory and practice without simply manipulating yoga so that it conveniently fits into our lifestyle. Yoga does not offer consolation or security through blind faith or elaborate theories of god, fantasies of a better afterlife or safety in the face of death. Rather, yoga teaches us to value our existential disorientation and to look into it deeply and without distraction.

In order to be truly free, you must desire to know the truth more than you want to feel good. Practicing in a way that supports our lifestyle and everything we already know is not a challenge to our basic patterns of conditioning in body, mind, and heart, because if feeling good is our goal, then as soon as we feel better, we will lose interest in what is true. Yoga is the union underneath good and bad, heaven and hell, self and no self; a set of practices aimed at the resolution of opposites. This does not mean that feeling good or experiencing joy or bliss is a bad thing. Given the choice, anyone would choose to feel bliss rather than sorrow. It simply means that if the desire to feel good is stronger than the yearning to see, know, and experience reality honestly, then this desire will always be distorting the perception of what is real while corrupting one's deepest integrity. Yoga is the natural state of being with what is, and practice supports us in waking up to this natural state. The important point, though, is that we need practice, practical tools, and everyday skills that help us move outside of our conditioned patterns, and for this we need some kind of system. But the system is not the yoga, only the technology for waking us up to the inherent interpermeation of existence.

If the true teacher is the present moment, everything is practice. However, we need some formal practice in order to learn the skills necessary to actually interrupt the momentum of distraction and wandering. That is why we have to practice yoga postures with great concentration, patience, grace, and subtlety. That is why we practice sitting meditation with pure acceptance and curious investigation. That is why we try always to refine our insight into impermanence, the contingency of self-image, the transience of all things, and the ways in which we create our own duḥkha. In the second chapter of the *Yoga-Sutra,* while discussing clinging as a case of mistaken fixation, Patañjali prescribes a complete reversal of perception as the necessary route out of ignorance: "Lacking this wisdom, one mistakes that which is impermanent, impure, distressing, or empty of self, for permanence, purity, happiness and self."[5]

The present moment is very easy to talk about, and when someone can speak about it clearly, we get a taste of waking up. Many of us feel this way after reading books about yoga or attending workshops. We go on retreat and return home only to find that within a few days many of our deepest habits continue to surface. Habits always have momentum. That is why we need more than books or momentary insight. We need to embody the technology of waking up as more than a skill set and certainly as more than a new philosophy so that it becomes a way of being fully in life, and over time such an approach to practice will generate communities of practitioners and a culture focused on genuine freedom and care for one another.

Our insights need to be tested out over and over again in varying contexts. Practice and community are essential for this. Maybe some are born into a very awake existence, and Patañjali states that this is the case, but I know that, for me, the present is conceptual without the grounding of practice. "Practice, practice, practice," says Pattabhi Jois, "and all is coming."

I would add to Pattabhi Jois's statement that when practice is grounded in theory and theory in practice, our insight becomes not just deep but wide. Over time, awareness touches everything, like crisscrossing lines stretched out over everything. When practice and theory go together seamlessly and our insights are continually tested out in real life, our waking up is practical and ongoing. This is called *prajña* (wisdom). Wisdom is the testing out, refinement, and maturation of insight. A practice that matures, both by working with the mind-body process but also through expression in community, leads to a life of wisdom. Marcel Proust sums up the cultivation of wisdom as follows:

> We do not receive wisdom, we must discover it for ourselves, after a journey through the wilderness, which no one else can make for us, which no one can spare us, for our wisdom is the point of view from which we come at last to regard the world.[6]

Yoga is concerned with opening up our ways of regarding and acting in the world. Beginning in the body, yoga teaches us how to discover for ourselves the inherent unity of life. Free from doctrine and certainly from dogma, we are asked to wake up to the reality of being present in an ever-changing world without clinging to anything as "I, me, or mine." This is the heart of practice. This is the heart of nonduality. An internal or psychological approach to yoga uses perception in this very moment as the path that leads toward waking up from the dualistic habits of clinging and repetitiveness. Practice that includes the psychological aspects of waking up teaches us how to interrupt the momentum of past conditioning in order to lead a life of ongoing awakening. Stephen Batchelor writes,

> By paying mindful attention to the sensory immediacy of experience, we realize how we are created, moulded, formed

> by a bewildering matrix of contingencies that continually arise and vanish. On reflection, we see how we are formed from the patterning of the DNA derived from our parents, the firing of a hundred billion neurons in our brains, the cultural and historical conditioning of the twentieth century, the education and upbringing given us, all the experiences we have ever had and choices we have ever made. These processes conspire to configure the unrepeatable trajectory that culminates in this present moment. What is here now is the unique but shifting impression left by all of this, which I call "me."
>
> Moreover, this gradual dissolution of a transcendental basis for self nurtures an empathetic relationship with others. The grip of self not only leads to alienation but numbs one to the anguish of others. Heartfelt appreciation of our own contingency enables us to recognize our inter-relatedness with other equally contingent forms of life. We find that we are not isolated units but participants in the creation of an ongoing, shared reality.[7]

Our practice, like our lives, does not arrive fully unfolded. Our work is to practice in such a way that makes sense for our particular life but also challenges the stories of ourselves that enclose our lives in cycles of habit. With clarity, flexibility, and steadiness, yoga teaches us how to move responsively through the details of life. This is possible in every unfolding moment of reality. Adyanshanti writes,

> To the extent that the fire of truth wipes out all fixated points of view, it wipes out inner contradictions as well, and we begin to move in a whole different way. The Way is the flow that comes from a place of non-contradiction—not from good and bad. Much less damage tends to be done from that place. Once we have reached the phase where there is no fixed self-

> concept, we tend to lead a selfless life. The only way to be selfless is to be self less—without a self. No matter what it does, a self isn't going to be selfless. It can pretend. It can approximate selflessness, but a self is never going to be selfless because there is always an identified personal self at the root of it.[8]

Such an attitude creates in practitioners an ongoing evaluation of and commitment to our practice until the distinctions between formal and informal practice begin to dissolve, as do the frames that create any form of separation. Eventually we come to see that we penetrate the mysteries of being simply by letting go into the mystery itself. There is nothing more infinite than this very moment, which is exactly where yoga begins.

# 19. *Śūnyatā:*

## BOUNDLESS AND EMPTY

Beyond the senses are the objects,
Beyond the objects is the mind,
Beyond the mind, the intellect,
Beyond the intellect, the ātman,
Beyond the ātman, the non-manifest,
Beyond the non-manifest, the spirit,
Beyond the spirit there is nothing,
This is the end, pure awareness.

—*Katha Upaniṣad*

THE LANGUAGE to which traditional yoga practices belong speaks in terms of the "self," "soul," "spirit," and "seer." However, those terms are used much differently than they are in Western culture, and over thousands of years great care has been taken to define and redefine them in the light of deep meditative practices. Yoga practice has always moved hand in hand with a constant refinement of language. In most meditative traditions, teachers have taken great care with the language that they use to describe their experience, because language always captures our experience within borders that are too limited.

*Śūnyatā* is an example of a term close to the heart of Patañjali but most associated with the teaching of the Buddha. However, we also find the term *śūnya* repeated in Patañjali's *Yoga-Sutra* many times and at key moments. Recent scholarship shows the roots of the *Yoga-Sutra* drawing from the teachings of the Buddha, yet irrespective of these traditional ties, the teaching of śūnyatā has specific meanings in the context of yoga psychology. What the Buddha and Patañjali share is the distrust of leaning on the names we have for clear, unmodified awareness. When one has an experience of being completely open and transparent, the mind automatically wants to name it.

The Indologist R. C. Zaehner, in a text on mysticism dating from 1957, characterizes the difficulty in conceiving the teachings on pure awareness found in Patañjali's *Yoga-Sutra* when he says that yoga has "perhaps the strangest conception of 'God' known to the whole of religion."[1] Again, yoga sidesteps the issue of blind faith in God by offering practical techniques for liberation matched with a distrust in reifying our experience with language and concepts.

At first, the Hindu way of talking about the phenomenon of complete and unmediated reality seems diametrically opposed to what one finds in Buddhism. In the same way someone interested in the theory of Carl Jung would do well to begin with Sigmund Freud, it is important to explore the *Yoga-Sutra* in the context of the Sāṇkhya, Hindu, and Buddhist systems that predate it. The Hindu description of *jīva,* the Advaita description of *ātman-brahman,* and the Buddhist notion of no-self or emptiness seem at odds with one another. Are they not just ways of talking about the same experience? It would be unwise to simplify these traditions and say they are talking about the same thing only in different languages, because that would deny the uniqueness of each system. But what is interesting about the *Yoga-Sutra* is that it teaches that pure awareness (puruṣa) is empty of self (*sva*) and form (*rūpa*), which places Patañjali's teaching square in the middle of these diametrically opposed ways of talking about reality. Patañjali's teachings on *svarūpa śūnya* slide in between the Hindu and Buddhist doctrines by giving a name to awareness and then turning the name inside out. This paradox urges us to think deeply about the language we use to talk about reality.

This naming is harmless on first impression, because it creates a context for understanding, whatever way that context fits our worldview: God, Self, Jesus, Emptiness, and so on. But the Buddha and Patañjali both push the limits farther by using the idea of "śūnya" not as a final place or resting point or ontological axiom but rather as a means for seeing how our use of language restricts and shuts down experience by reifying it. Language is the framework within which we render our experience meaningful. We represent our experience through language. We refract and embody our experience with words and ideas. The words and ideas are usually grounded in some faith that something about this path we are embarking on is going to offer some peace, some kind of transformation, and the words become clusters of assumptions, expectation, and cultural representations of the mystical experience. When we have a direct experience of being present, it is usually interrupted by a mind that comes in and says "I am completely present." The mind always comes in and uses language and cultural symbols to articulate the experience of nonduality. The problem is that when the experience is articulated, we are pulled out of it.

Even when we use the word *emptiness,* we often think of a void or the experience of no-self. We also associate the terms *emptiness* and *no-self* with a distinctly Buddhist context. But these terms are used in yoga in similar ways, and though often misunderstood or avoided altogether, they have compelling and practical value and are important to consider in the context of the yoga path. One can also translate *śūnyatā* as "boundlessness," or "that which has no borders." The job of language, like the job of yoga itself, is to create and enlarge a true understanding of oneself and the nature of reality. Terms such as *śūnyatā,* or even terms like *soul* or *god,* are only useful inasmuch as they are treated as tools rather than as the final end point of doctrine. The poet Rainer Maria Rilke, in an inscription he put into the copy of *Duino Elegies* that he gave to his Polish translator, writes,

Happy are those who know:
Behind all words, the Unsayable stands;
And from that source, the Infinite
Crosses over to gladness, and us.

Free of those bridges we raise
With constructed distinctions;
So that always, in each separate joy,
We gaze at the single, wholly mutual core.[2]

Emptiness is not the negation or elimination of a sense of self, but paradoxically the state of being in one's true nature. Although we give privileged significance to the term *emptiness,* in the same way that we do with terms like *samādhi* or *enlightenment,* emptiness is actually a tool, a strategy, rather than a final state. Emptiness is not a holy utopia, it is simply a way of describing a letting go, a loss, a falling away of that which keeps us separate from others, the world, and even ourselves. Emptiness is a tool we use that cuts away clinging, especially to our notions of a solid and substantial world, and thus a solid sense of "me" at the center of that world. What is the center of the world other than our idea that there is a recognizable center?

> There was neither non-existence nor existence then. . . . There was neither death nor immortality then. There was no distinguishing sign of night nor of day.[3]

The *Rig-Veda* goes on in humbling paradox:

> Who really knows? . . . The gods came afterwards with the creation of the universe. Who then knows whence it has arisen?[4]

The hymn then concludes with a more astonishing question:

> Whence this creation has arisen—perhaps it formed itself—or perhaps it did not—the one who looks down on it, in the highest heaven, only he knows—or perhaps he does not know.[5]

"Perhaps he does not know" ends the debate with a question allowed to be left as a question. How flexible, one might add, to allow the central axiom of your metaphysical system and worldview to be nothing other than the questioning of your basic questions. This is not pluralism but rather a very deep insight into the psychology of belief, the basis of our faith. Since what we believe determines the kind of world we perceive and the kinds of actions we take, if we multiply our belief systems by zero (śūnya), we arrive in an open field of perception.

When the Upaniṣads later comment on the Vedas, and the reader is asked once again to consider whether the ultimate reality is "this" or "that," the Upaniṣads respond with *neti, neti* (not like this, not like that). Great suffering is accrued by attachment to views, and when we cut into the heart of our psychology, we find at the base of things attachment to views. Perspectives on all matters of life, from "who am I" to "how did this begin" and "how and where will it end," are valuable as instrumental questions to work with, but the answers derived from such questions are not to be venerated in and of themselves. So in what state of mind do we want to move through the world today?

Emptiness as a tool assists us in removing that which cuts us off from the web of life we are immersed in. *Emptiness* is a utilitarian term, not a description of a sacred space or a claim of truth. It is about creating space in our relationship to ourselves, through which we can free the mind from fixations that isolate and reduce us to the claims of an isolated and self-referential ego. When there is space, we find ourselves in the midst of life rather than entangled in a solipsistic experience of self around which life pivots. Svarūpa śūnya is a teaching or strategy that aims to dismantle our belief in the substantiality of what we perceive, especially the belief that at the center of the personality is a substantial or essential "me."

Yet this "me" is a holdover, conceptually speaking, from the past. It is not untrue that there is a self-referential mechanism in the mind, but what is untrue is its permanence and substantiality. Past and present as noticed in the mind are just mind states of past and present. This shows us that at the heart of the world, in the center of our conception of our personality, at the base of our worldviews and metaphysical stories, we find a reality not bound by our stories and ideas. We find at the center of reality, a reality without edges, boundless, and by definition centerless.

Before our son was born, my partner and I had a few ideas for names. Once he was born, it seemed somehow obvious that one of the names we had in mind, Arlyn, would fit well. It was exciting giving this new creature, this new person, a name. Yet it also felt odd adding a name to the emerging life that we had just created. Yet conventionally a name seemed appropriate. For the first few days I couldn't get used to it. It wasn't the particular name we had chosen; rather it was the fact that we were overlaying this new baby with a fixed term. He was not his name.

When you ask yourself the question, who am I?, if you can allow yourself to observe what happens from a place of stillness, you can see how self-constructed our ideas of self are. When we can probe the thoughts and feelings and sense of self that arise from asking this question, the less it becomes possible to identify anything in the changing field of perception as "me." Is the breath mine? Am I the one who breathes? Who is that? Are sounds mine? Is the ear mine? Are feelings in the body mine? Is the body mine?

In a conventional sense it is of course important to have a sense of who I am and where I begin and others end. But this is a malleable and fluid definition. I need to know who I am as opposed to who you are, or my psychological world will be in chaos. Through influences that we have come in contact with and choices that we made in past experiences, and also through biology and what we have inherited, we all have unique characteristics. These characteristics, in a relative sense, define us.

But we tend to cluster around that identity and think of it as something separate and apart. In meditation, through exploring the nature of each moment, we begin to see that what we thought was rigid and solid is actually impermanent and interdependent. The concrete sense of "I" begins to break down. It becomes increasingly difficult to pinpoint anything—a feeling, perception, sensation, thought—as essentially "me."

We might ask this of Patañjali when he describes the technique of *dharma megha samādhi.* In meditation practices, he suggests, one finds a field in which the building blocks of our experience are seen to be impermanent, in constant flux. He says, "One can see that the flow [of reality] is actually a series of discreet events, each corresponding to the merest instance of time, in which one form becomes another."[6]

When we see that the fundamental qualities of nature are always changing and that anything that is perceivable is also changing, how is it possible to fix one of those points and call it "me"? Emptiness is the "unfindability" of things. It is the almost infinite depth when you begin to probe into the questions of who am I? what am I? what is this? No matter how deeply and acutely you search for "me" in mind and body, it escapes investigation. If the mind as a microscope looks for the essence of "me," it will result in loss. But this loss is revealing—it is the opening in the fabric of life of a path or dimension that is not something and also not nothing. In fact there is no-thing to be found. So what at first seems like loss becomes something to cultivate. Emptiness is not found as void or as nothing, but it is also not found as something.

This may seem confusing at first, but emptiness is a tool designed to dislodge the tendency in the mind toward reification—the belief that things are substantial, real, and reliable. It's an opening up to the experience that the "I", the body, or even the mind, is not reducible to something. Probing does not mean we arrive at no-thing. In yoga we always move from that which is known to that which is unknown. We use the known in order to find its edges. At the edges of the known, life reveals itself, because we have arrived at the limits of knowledge, the limits of understanding.

We move in the body in this way also—from comfortable ways of walking and talking toward that which is outside of habitual parameters.

We begin looking into what is known about the body or the breath, and when we push it further, such as when we hold a posture for an extended period of time, we lose our sense of it, only to have a direct experience of the posture. We use the form of the posture to experience śūnyatā, boundlessness. Śūnyatā is freedom beyond the reach of karma, a body beyond the reach of preference, movement without self-image. Isn't the experience of simply being alive in a body at all the most mysterious and ineffable experience we can know? We use yoga postures to wake up the five *buddhindriyas* (sense capacities): hearing, feeling, seeing, tasting, and smelling; as well as the five corresponding *karmedriyas* (action capacities): speaking, holding, walking, excreting, and procreating; along with the five *tanmātras* (subtle material elements) as sensed by the mind-body: sound, touch, form, taste, and smell.

These capacities, actions, and material elements are all products of the five *mahābhūtas* (gross material elements): space, wind, fire, water, air, and earth. Whether from a cosmological or an individual perspective, consciousness is intimately tied up with the body, which is dependent for its existence on the basic constituent elements in nature.

The more that we look at the primary constituents of mental and physical experience, like a scientist studying the substratum of matter, we certainly don't arrive at a final conclusion, but we also don't dissolve into nothingness. Every layer of reality that we explore reveals yet another layer, more nuanced, complex, and mysterious. We look deeply into the breath and we find the air element, and when there is a release in a breathing pattern, we immediately sense space. We study muscles, and fascia is revealed. We study fascia, and other physical holding patterns are revealed. We study physiology, and psychology is revealed, and we study psychology, and the nature of mind is revealed. This process keeps going and going, and the deeper we investigate, the closer we come to unraveling the mystery of life and its processes. The more we look at something, the less know about it. We are confronted at every turn of experience not with hard facts but with the possibility of intimacy. When we become intimate with what we perceive, we experience life unmediated by the hardened narrative of self. Then we find ourselves open to an otherness that is no longer outside of our experience but right at the heart of pure being: we experience how the body is a conglomeration of conditions, including mind and breath, that has nothing at all to do with self-image. At last we come to the heart of yoga—an intimacy in which we find ourselves in the vast circle of life, cherishing all aspects of life equally and committed to the renewal of our best resources: awareness, kindness, and loving action.

## *Hands Down*

We plant our hands on the earth in Downward-Facing Dog pose, fingers outstretched like giant webs supporting elevated hips and long legs. Think about the number of times you have practiced Downward-Facing Dog pose. At first, as beginners, we suffer through the posture, simply learning how to put our hands squarely on the yoga mat as we exhale and lift our pelvis away from the floor. Then as we learn more techniques and the body becomes accustomed to the posture, we find comfort or relative stability in the pose. But as we delve deeper into the pose, perhaps several decades later, the posture becomes mysterious again.

I recall studying once with Richard Freeman where at the start of the ten-day session we explored Downward-Facing Dog. We explored the pose for a whole morning until all of our thoughts about Downward-Facing Dog became irrelevant. Over and over, we went deeper and deeper into the pose until we were in the posture with no ideas about it. Just pure experience. On the last day of this ten-day session, he returned again to Downward Dog. All afternoon we explored the pose over and over until the entire workshop dissolved into immediate physical experience. The mind had no ideas about the posture anymore. The mind and body were like one big question mark. How can we continually practice like this, turning the mind and body into a process rather than a system of knowledge, always questioning, always inquiring within?

Inquiry is infinite. Emptiness is the infinite nature of inquiry. Emptiness is emptying, a releasing of certain attachments. What are we emptying ourselves of? What we are letting go is our bias and perspective. It's not simply letting go of a perspective in the way we might let go of a cherished idea, though that is helpful. Letting go of our perspective means letting go of a particular hold or grip we have on something. It is not perspective or viewpoint that is the problem but how tightly we hold on to that perspective. So the key here is seeing a perspective as simply a perspective. A view is always one of an infinite number of views, though usually it feels like we hold on to to one without looking at the huge number of perspectives always available to us.

Moving beyond the personal perspective of "I, me and mine" reveals that which is awake, present, and beyond words. Here is an exchange between the nondual teacher Sri Nisargadatta Maharaj and a visitor:

> Maharaj: As a matter of fact, mind is a universal dynamic principle, but we restrict it to the limits of the body and then depend on it—hence all the trouble. Consider the water in Lake Tansa. That water belongs to the whole of Bombay. Out of that water, can we claim some as yours or mine? In a similar vein, understand that the self is universal. But you have conditioned it by confining it to the body; therefore, you face problems. This self is also termed Ishvara—God—the Universal Principle. If you hold on to that, profound knowledge will descend upon you and you will have peace.

Visitor: I try to meditate on that, but the mind wanders here and there. If I try to remain indifferent to mind, it will be a long-drawn-out process.

Maharaj: But are you not the root of any process?

Visitor: The root of everything is life.

Maharaj: Yes, but the life force is universal and not personalized. Once you realize this, you have no more troubles.[7]

Grasping is the root of what eventually becomes a belief or an opinion. Trying to hold on to to something fixed and stable in the midst of an impermanent and fluctuating world creates duḥkha. Grasping feels as though it is not a mental or physical choice but somehow instinctual as a survival mechanism. It comes with the biological organism. Perhaps ancient Indian thought did not have the ideas of biology we have now, but there seems to be the idea that we drop into the world with the tendency toward grasping.

Recently I was offering some banana to our son. He was sitting up in his high chair devouring the banana and asking for more. I got up to get another banana and then looked back at his smiling and insatiable grin. He has huge Dizzy Gillespie cheeks. He had banana in his right cheek, banana in his left cheek, banana all over his face, and his hands were oozing with banana. He had banana all over his table, and still he wanted more banana. Since his mouth was full, he couldn't even say so, but the look in his eyes forecasted a desire for even more banana. Although it's easy to idealize the goal of yoga as being able to be as present as a child, we forget sometimes that kids come into the world with a great deal of clinging. We are born clinging.

That is why yoga is not about setting up a new belief system, of emptiness for example, but using the teaching to learn about how we grasp. Then we use the techniques offered by yoga to let go. We tend to separate life into categories and concepts that create a fragmented and split experience. This is natural and may not be bad thing in and of itself, but we don't see and certainly don't realize that these splits are conceptual categories. Though this is a necessary function and social device, it leads us to a fictional sense of who we are and what is real. Fixity equals closure; closure inevitably becomes inflexibility.

The debate about yoga, Hinduism, and Buddhism often becomes focused around the definition of self. On first appearance the Buddhist notion of not-self contradicts the Hindu teaching on ātman and Brahman, the essential self. But on closer investigation, the pre-Buddhist "self" is not what one thinks; it's beyond linguistic conceptualization and has no form or qualities. The teachings on emptiness or ātman are strategies rather than final metaphysical truths. When we treat these concepts as strategies, we avoid the pitfall of confusing a technique with fantasies of ultimate truth. The theologian Don Cupitt writes,

> Of these fixed points, the idea of the Self is one of the most important. We want to imagine that there is a Real Me, a substance, something enduring and self-identical in us that transcends the flux of life. However, for so long as we believe in any fixed points outside the flux of life, we will be incapable of Glory and afraid of death. Life is outsideless. Glory means giving up all ideas of substance, all absolutes and things outside time, and losing our Selves in the flux of life. Jesus seems to compare "eternal life" with the way birds and flowers live, meaning that if we who are spirit can achieve the same exact coincidence with our own pure contingency that comes so naturally to the lily and the bird, then, we shall have eternal life. Death's sting is drawn.[8]

Even yoga texts such as the *Yoga Vāsiṣṭa* describe this paradox without clinging to a final view on the matter: "Awareness of course has no distinct form.... It is known as the mind, the true self or emptiness."[9]

We can always set up a vocabulary that names experience in different ways—as sacred, divine, soul, spirit, self—but these distinctions are mere appearances, not the actuality of insight or wisdom, and always come after the facts of experience. In essence these are just words to describe an experience that cannot be described with words. The ultimate truth of things is timeless, but it is a truth rooted in human experience, not a holy book or mystical system someone far away achieved in a culture now unknown to us. In order for a teaching to be of liberative value, it has to be known in the life of you and me. Yoga has to be known and absorbed directly. That is why we begin by always turning the mind to such simple objects: the breath at this moment, the body as it's felt at this moment. All of the advanced techniques of yoga are right here in these two simple methods: breathing your circumstances, staying in the body. Nobody can do this for us.

When the mind, body, and nervous system settle down and interest in the investigation of experience increases, inner and outer life open up in greater degrees of texture and detail. Yet the mind still tries to grasp after finality or certainty. The next stage of practice is the gradual development of wisdom (*prajña).* Wisdom is the ability to suspend knowledge (*jñāna*) and is the antidote to the distortions and illusions that plant most of the seeds of suffering. Wisdom, in the context of the kleṣas, is the embodied understanding of the unsatisfactoriness of whatever is impermanent and the way we are driven by attachment to pleasure (raga) and aversion (dveṣa) to what is not pleasurable. Wisdom is also knowing the extent to which self-identity is manufactured and then projected onto all experience, and the way this "self" construction hinders a spontaneous and ethical response to life and the great questions it presents. We have a moral obligation to wake up.

# 20. Yoga, Death, and Dying

## WHAT IS MOST ASTOUNDING?

IN THE EPIC Indian story called the *Mahābhārata,* the sage Yuddhiṣṭhira is asked, "Of all things in life, what is the most astounding?" Yuddhiṣṭhira responds, "That a person, seeing others die all around him, never thinks that he will die."

Aging is an opportunity to develop one's curiosity regarding the course of life this body takes. One of the deepest pains of being human is the realization that every aspect of life is undergoing constant change and that everything once born is then subject to decay and death. What becomes a singular life also passes away, and in this way the singular is seen to be part of a much larger, pulsing whole. And each body in contact with its environment runs a specific course, a unique path of aging. There is a primary unwillingness, especially in our culture, to look at aging directly. To be accepting of aging and dying brings us face-to-face with our ongoing and unconscious repression of the awareness of death and dying.

Yoga demands that we look the serpent right in the mouth until we realize it has no poison. We can be present even when death squeezes the last exhalation from the body. It is through a deep investigation of what it means to be structured in a life of impermanence and provisionality that we are moved to open fully to the reality of what is our everyday, every-moment experience. In the face of death, there is nothing left to avoid and certainly nothing left to hold on to. There is a wonderful story in the *Srimad Bhagavatam,* a collection of eighteen thousand verses about the lives of avatars, yogis, sages, and kings, in which the sage Narada teaches a very basic truth to a confused king:

> "All worldly identifications and all attachments that pass as relationships are fraught with sorrow. All relationships are conceptual. They appear and disappear like a palace in the clouds. On account of inherent tendencies that come to life at birth, people think of all objects, relationships and selves as real and indulge in action rooted in this ignorance."

The king, confused by these assertions, responds by asking Narada why people keep clinging and how to overcome these attachments and delusions. Narada responds,

> "The one direct cause for people's sorrow is their deluded sense that the body is the self. One clings to the body as one's own. Correct and diligent investigation into the nature of the self is the only sure cure for this malady."

On hearing this, the king regains his balance of mind. He realizes that what he was most attached to was his sense of self and his identification with his body, and that as long as he identified the impermanent body as being owned by his own sense of self, he remained outside of reality because he thought of others as separate.[1]

The "I" has nothing to cling to, because all experiences are impermanent. This is most easily observed by watching the sensations in the body come and go or thoughts in the mind appear and disappear. Yoga reminds us that, having been born, we are subject to aging and inevitable death. We might avoid old age, some of us might not get sick, but the body will die sooner or later. Although we know this, the only thing we cannot know is where or when, and life becomes a coming together and coming apart of an ongoing matrix of conditions, intertwined and mysterious, like scaffolds on scaffolds, flowers from seeds, atoms dancing.

There is not much incentive in contemporary culture to contemplate our own mortality. When someone becomes sick or dies, it is a chance for us to recognize that this can happen to us at any time. In the yoga tradition, the teachings ask a basic question: If death is inevitable, why wait until the last moments of life to contemplate death? Why not in this moment? This is why we practice *savāsanā* (Corpse pose), or as Pattabhi Jois says, "Practicing death, little bit every day."

Aging and death bring urgency to practice. If the time of death does come soon, what will I regret that I had not done? How would I have wanted to live my life? Am I living my life fully? Do I use every moment as something I can learn from?

When my friend, who is struggling with cancer, described her recent chemotherapy session, she said,

> Many people assume that the experience of cancer is overwhelmingly negative, and many people living with cancer feel that their experience of cancer should conform to this concept of negativity. Yes, cancer and the treatment for it can be terrible. But cancer is also amazing because to say that cancer is only terrible is to separate it from all of life that surrounds it. The beautiful people you meet in waiting rooms, the support and generosity of family and friends, the diligent and thoughtful care by so many professionals, the unique opportunity for reflection and contemplation—there is an entire experience of life while we are experiencing cancer. When we say cancer is terrible, where does cancer the terrible end, and all these wonderful side effects we call life begin? All of life with cancer is cancer, and all of cancer is life. Cancer and life

> are not separate and not distinct. So we can't categorize our experience. We can just experience it for what it is.[2]

This also helps us appreciate one another in a very different way. With mindfulness there is a resolution to be more sensitive, more careful. It's like when we drive in the snow, we take greater care. We don't get frustrated with the fact of the snow. The snow comes whether we want it to or not. All we can do is take great care with how we drive. We see the snow as an incentive to be present, mindful, and fully aware.

It's much easier to evaluate experience than it is to accept it. Even in subtle ways, it is hard to allow each moment to be full or enough. Even to let ourselves be ourselves, acting without a persona or attachment, simply being for the sake of being. Isn't the heart of acceptance rooted in our own hearts? What would it mean to accept every aspect of ourselves? In the contemplation of death we come to see that we don't need to get things right anymore; instead we can begin to accept each moment just as it is. We can let others be as others are.

Often when we hear of acceptance, we think of surrender or sacrifice. But nothing is unacceptable. Even the greatest suffering in the wider world or the strongest currents of pain within ourselves can be accepted. Acceptance doesn't mean liking something or agreeing with it. It is rather an allowing. Not shutting things out. Yoga is the practice of allowing things to be as they are and not turning away from any part of reality. If I am in a situation I can't bear, then it is the unbearable that is to be accepted.

By accepting our aging just as it is, we allow for all that we are. Be with your experience directly. How do you do that? Awareness simply reflects what is there. It reveals all that is there without comment or comparison. In aging and illness, even in pain, we notice how we react in each moment. Are we holding on? Are we pushing away? How does this moment feel in the body? Are we contracting or pulling away? When there is contraction, we can't see clearly.

Contraction denotes turning away. We don't need to make aging or illness any different. We can be with the state of what is actually present, even if it is fear, pain, or despair, if we can give that state space without turning from it. When we contract, we cannot possibly notice how things are because we are blocking out our experience at both a sensual and a mental level.

We don't need to make this body any different—that is the practice of *satya* (honesty) with the body—we see this aging body for what it is. We can be with the mind state that is there without trying to create a new one. If we can give a state space rather than struggling with it, things begin to settle down on their own. The energy that was defending against what was unfolding in awareness can be freed up. When everything is seen clearly, it is easier to act wisely and accept the reality of our circumstances. Liberation from delusion means precisely the release of our energies of death denial. The repression of our awareness of impermanence eventually yields a release of our strategies against death's arrival. The symptoms of such repression manifest in us as a deep and outward need for security. Whether we seek the material security of capital, the relational security of romantic love, the ego's security in fame and notoriety, it really makes no difference. All of the symptoms of attachment and aversion come down to the basic denominator of impermanence that reminds us that all concrete embodiments in any sphere across any species are structured within a limited time span.

No matter how fixed and concrete they appear on the surface, mind states, like the ongoing sensations of the body, are always loosening and passing away. The *Ashtavakra Gītā,* one of the many anonymous Indian teachings or folk tales known as *purāṇas,* describes this with great clarity:

> All things arise,
> Suffer change,
> And pass away.

This is their nature.

When you know this . . .<br>
. . . you become still.<br>
It is easy.[3]

In practice we are including rather than excluding. We expend so much energy avoiding the way life actually unfolds, and most of the time we are not aware that we doing this. This is exhausting. When we begin to see that there can be spaciousness where there was resistance, the contents of consciousness gain less of a purchase on us. Each time we make space, trust grows. The more we trust reality, the more the mind's habits of aversion lose their footing.

Trusting in this practice is a form of training the heart. Being interested in yoga is being interested in the heart and its opening. Most of us have been through enough suffering, joy, and the range of emotions in between to know that unless there is a context for our experience, it doesn't lead anywhere. Sometimes I think practice is a way of setting life in context, and certainly many of our psychological ills are more meaningful and manageable when seen in the context of spiritual practice. With a context it becomes more than chaos or more than a routine without solace. The heart knows that life is more than that, and paradoxically this provokes the ego into a kind of anxiousness because when we see the self is a changing and impermanent mechanism rather than an ongoing "thing" in space and time, we see that anxiety is central to the ego, because it is the self's response to its own groundlessness.

The heart is not just a location or an intellectual place but rather the greater part of us, and it has the ability to feel freedom within changing conditions. As a metaphor in yoga terminology and physiology, the heart is bright and peaceful, but only because it is "unstruck" by the reality of change. What creates our "problems" is the way that we identify with and cling to that which moves through the heart. Identification is the root of clinging. If you understand that, you find the heart of practice. If there is clinging, there is dissatisfaction, and if there is no clinging, there is no suffering. In one of his last poems, entitled "Late Fragment," Raymond Carver offers this truth in concise terms:

> And did you get what
> You wanted from this life, even so?
> I did.
> And what did you want?
> To call myself beloved, to feel myself
> Beloved on the earth.[4]

When we practice sincerely, what we want in life becomes simpler and simpler. What yoga teaches us is to stop looking outside the heart for satisfaction. We are so clever at finding external reasons to perpetuate our habits, because even if we see that our habits cause us distress, we keep repeating them because they are known. This is why we practice. Time by itself does not heal these kinds of illusions. If they are not seen directly, time just entrenches them further. We need a strong commitment to letting go and to paying attention to the clinging involved in difficult mental and physical states. Accepting aging and death is a good start.

When we inspect our everyday experience in detail, we see that death and birth occur one after the other in every successive moment. What we see in one breath cycle we see everywhere. Just as a scientist who studies interdependence cannot bring an entire ecosystem into a laboratory, we cannot, on the surface, examine all of the facets of existence at once. However, when you focus intently without too many preconceptions on something as simple as the breath or the changing (*pariṇāma*) sensations in the body—what Patañjali calls dharma megha samādhi—we get a sense of the truths of existence, especially the truth of change. When we inspect our moment-to-moment experience, we find we are not permanent objects or selves but perceptual elements coming together and coming apart. Some schools of yoga refer to this as "the *gunas*"—the changing particles that make up the substratum of experience. But there is nothing gluing this ebb and flow together except the ability to see these patterns as ebbing and flowing—what comes together always comes apart. All the basic patterns, constituents, or elements in nature come together and come apart. There is nothing to hold on to and nothing to which we can ascribe selfhood. These building blocks, like atoms, are not "things" that exist but rather the smallest particles of perception available to us. If you look at one moment of sensation in the body, for example, you can see it as a constantly changing configuration of elements.

Anyone who has spent time with the dying knows how life-affirming a close experience of dying can be. And as far as we know, nobody has been able to escape death. Of the current world population of over five billion people, almost none will be alive in a hundred years' time. Not only do our thoughts, relationships, and bodies have a time limit, so do our conceptions of ourselves. We are in constant motion. Life has a definite, inflexible limit, and each moment brings us closer to its finality. We are dying from the moment we are born.

Impermanence also teaches us that death comes in a moment and that its time is unexpected. All that separates us from the next life is one breath. When we are born, our first autonomous gesture after leaving the womb is our first inhale. When we die, we leave the world on an exhale. In between, however, the duration of our life span is uncertain. The young can die before the old, the healthy before the sick. The physical body contributes to life's seeming certainty, but its weakness and fragility also reveal its uncertainty.

Worldly possessions can't help our position in the face of death and dying. Relatives and friends can neither prevent death nor go with us. Even our own precious body is of no help to us. We have to leave it behind like a shell, an empty husk, an overcoat. The form of the body will eventually come apart, like a seed fallen from a tree, and come together again under different conditions in yet another form.

In yoga practice, as we become more and more familiar with the patterns and movements of the breath and the other elements as well, we come into contact with the basic constituents of our experience. The basic elements of reality are called by various names in different systems—*gunas, kośas, skandhas, prakṛti, prāṇa vāyuu*—all with the same purpose, namely, to offer us tools or strategies we can use to meditate upon and eventually accept the changing reality in which we find ourselves. We see in the elements no place to cling and nowhere to identify an "I, me, or mine." This process of meditation teaches the practitioner the stages of death and the mind-body relationships behind them. The description of the dying process in most Indian texts is based on a presentation of the winds (vāyuu), or currents of energy, that serve as foundations for various levels of consciousness, and the channels in which they flow. Upon the serial collapse of the ability of these winds to serve as bases of consciousness, the internal and external events of death unfold. Through the power of meditation, the yogi makes the coarse winds dissolve into the very subtle life-bearing wind at the heart. This yoga mirrors the process that occurs at death and involves concentration on the psychic channels and their centers (chakras) inside the body.

At the chakras there are platforms upon which physical and mental health are based. The physiology of death revolves around changes in the winds and one's attitude in the process of dying. Since the mind is intimately linked with the winds of the breath, we watch them both. Psychologically, due to the fact that consciousnesses of varying grossness and subtlety depend on the winds, like a rider on a horse, their dissolving or loss of ability to serve as bases of consciousness induces radical changes in conscious experience.

Death begins with the sequential dissolution of the winds associated with the four elements (earth, water, fire, and air). "Earth" refers to the hard factors of the body, such as bone, and the dissolution of the wind associated with it means that that wind is no longer capable of serving as a mount or basis for consciousness. As a consequence of its dissolution, the capacity of the wind associated with "water" (the fluid factors of the body) to act as a mount for consciousness becomes more manifest. The ceasing of the capacity in one element and its greater manifestation in another is called "dissolution"—it is not, therefore, a case of gross earth dissolving into water. Simultaneous with the dissolution of the earth element, the other elements also begin to sequentially return to their respective base in the natural world.

All the elements can be found in any phenomenon in nature, whether internal or external. When one pays attention to the body in yoga posture practice, one is meditating on the elements. The earth element, much like the outer sheath of the first kośa, is characteristic of hardness, felt experience, heaviness, density, and defined space. As one begins dying, the bones become heavy, the skin pale, the eyes become difficult to open, and the sensory grasp of the world begins to slip away. As we meditate on the earth element in the form of the body, we feel the body slipping away, color withdrawing from the skin, and loss of control.

As the earth element transforms, we come into contact with the water element. Hearing begins to fade, the fluids of the body are out of our control, saliva drips from the mouth, water appears at the corners of the eyes, and it becomes difficult to hold urine. The lips become chapped, the nostrils cave into the septum, the eyes become very dry, and the fluids that characterize the water element dissolve into the fire element. Death chips away at everything.

The fire element withdraws and the body becomes cool and stiff, the breath becomes cold, the nose no longer smells scent, and digestion is no longer possible. As the characteristics of heat leave the body, we see signs of the dissolution of the air element as the out-breath grows longer and longer and the senses begin to fade away. Other people are no longer recognizable, there is no longer a sense of interest or purpose in the mind, and the ability to perceive begins to fade away completely. Death is always whispering a reminder, however quietly, that there is nothing at all we can cling to as ultimately mine; and in such awareness, life flows along transparently, a bankless stream.

When volition is completely given up, the dissolution of the air element becomes prominent; there is nowhere to go and nothing to do. The in-breath becomes shorter and shorter; the out-breath elongates and so does the pause at the bottom of each breath cycle. The pressures of meaning and purpose, the expectations of being somebody going somewhere, no longer trouble the mind. Gravity reigns over the body. Joan Halifax, in her research working with the dying, describes this process in detail:

> As the element of air is dissolved, you are having visions. Your visions may be jewellike and filled with insight that can never be expressed. These visions relate to who you are and how you have lived your life. You may be seeing your family or your ancestors in a peaceful setting. You may be seeing beautiful people, saints, or friends welcoming you. You may be reliving pleasant experiences from your past. Or you may have demonic and hellish visions. If you have hurt others, those whom you have injured may appear to you. Difficult and dreadful moments of your life may arise to haunt you. You may see people with whom you have had negative interactions attacking you. You may even cry out in fear. Do not identify with these visions. Simply let them be.[5]

The air element dissolves, and there is nothing left to do. Mental functioning comes to an end and so does consciousness. Consciousness dissolves into space, the last exhalation occurs, there is no sensation in the body, the element of wind dissolves completely. The kośas are extinguished and the elements of mind and body return to their source in the ongoing flux of nature.

We imagine this practice as a description of our own death so that we can release our own unique identity into the greater, ongoing universe. Returning these particles called "self" back to their source, even if we have no words for such a source, helps loosen our fixations and entanglements. It took the earth billions of years to establish itself, and here we are, moving about sustained by that billion-year evolution and eventually disappearing back into it. This is the greater evolution: continuity with the genetic and molecular functioning of this immense planetary system of which we are only a small part indeed. When teaching, I almost always read the instructions for dying or these descriptions of the elements during the ten minutes of savāsanā (Corpse pose) when the students are lying down, the room is dark, and the collective breath is coming into stillness. If not treated as a practice of dying, savāsanā is reduced to a relaxation exercise and divorced from its purpose as a meditation on impermanence and, by extension, gratitude.

The contemplation of impermanence and nonattachment, coupled with a meditation on the elements, is not only a meditation on finality—it is also a way of placing the practitioner of yoga in the midst of life. When we complete an exhalation or blink our eyes, this moment of experience is over. Every moment of perception passes away. Being present with the changing nature of reality is in itself a meditation on death, because we are being asked as practitioners to allow each and every moment to pass away. The Bhāgavata Purāṇa states:

> When, because of disease or advanced age, one is neither able to perform one's duties, study philosophy, or pursue spiritual knowledge, one should begin to fast. Properly placing the fires (of the body) within oneself and relinquishing the notion of "I" and "mine," one should then completely merge the aggregate elements into their causes. The knower of the self (should merge) the apertures of the body into space, the vital airs into the air, the heat into fire, the blood, phlegm

> and pus into water, and the rest into earth, from whence they came. One should place one's speech and subject matter of speaking into Agni, the two hands and their crafting capacity into Indra, the feet and their power of movement into Visnu, the Spirit of time, the genitals and sexual enjoyment into Prajapati, the anus and its power of evacuation into Mrtyu, directing each into their proper place. One should merge the sense of hearing, along with sound, in the directions, tactility with the sense of touch into the wind, and form along with vision, O King, into the sun. One should merge the tongue, along with the sense of taste, into water, and fragrance, along with the sense of smell, into earth. Mind, along with desires, into the Moon, intelligence, along with its objects, into the supreme seer (Brahma), actions and self-awareness into Rudra, from who proceeds the action of egotism and self-interest, existence and thought into the individual (knower of the field), and the individual along with the qualities of nature into the Supreme. Earth in water, water in fire, the latter in air, that into space, that into ego, and the latter into the totality of matter, that into the unmanifest, and that into the undying, imperishable. Thus, knowing the imperishable self to be made of consciousness without a second, one should come to an end, like a fire that has devoured its origins.[6]

This description of death practice leads to the separation of the elements. Traditionally one would meditate separately on each sentence in the aforementioned description not only at the end of life but as a daily meditation. This type of practice is found consistently in meditation-based religious traditions. As we know, when the elements separate, they then come back together in some different form. Molecules continue, water flows and evaporates and flows again. There is an elemental configuration of ourselves in all things. What dies?

Each aspect of life has an intrinsic value when we are paying attention. Each point in the infinitely broad net of Indra connects, mirrors, and is interdependent with all other points of reality. More intimate than sisters or brothers, each aspect of this wide and complex web of life supports and conditions the basic constituent pieces that, when assembled, feel like a self. Though hard to fathom and even harder to practice, there is a fundamental unity that connects not only parts of the body or parts of the mind but each of us to every living and nonliving particle of existence. Each part of this existence has a value as part of an ultimate reality. To let go of oneself in the fullness of the rain, in the pain of loss, in the joy of feeling met is to be part of this ultimate reality. Within change there is connection. Within the many there is one. There is nothing that stands between self and the world, even though on the surface the world often seems outside of our minds and bodies. But yoga teaches us that the world of the mind is the world of the body and that the two are neither two nor one. Enlightenment is not something someone hands to you atop a mountain or something you one day attain, but an offering of centerless responsiveness through the realization of who we truly are. Mokṣa, or true freedom, is the experience of an authorless life into and out of which all things are created and completed.

The term *mokṣa* originally referred to the last phase of an eclipse, where one body begins to move out of the shadow of another. In a solar eclipse, for example, when the moon and hidden sun start to draw away from one another, revealing again the blazing sun, darkness lifts and the two bodies move in their respective spheres. Like the last phase of an eclipse, *mokṣa* refers to the freedom that occurs when one creates the conditions in mind and body for the dissolution of the five kleṣas and the end of suffering. The radical theologian Don Cupitt writes,

> We seem to have forgotten how to die. We have come to equate religion with holding on, when we ought to have been learning to see religion as teaching us how to let go. Religious

> belief should be producing a self-emptying way of life: we live by dying, unattached, pouring ourselves out into the flux of life in such a way that death when it comes is not a threat but a consummation.
>
> We should live as the sun does. Its existence, the process by which it lives, and the process by which it dies, all exactly coincide. It believes nothing, it hasn't a care, it just pours itself out.[7]

When we give attention to the way the body and mind are made of elements, it becomes easy to see impermanence. When we pay attention to the way the elements come together and when we stay with the changing nature of each element in and of itself, it is hard to find anything to cling to as "I, me, or mine." This eliminates the delusion of our ordinary perceptual attitude that the body continues in space and time. This body is impermanent.

The only thing Patañjali says about the body at the time of death is as follows: "Once the body dies and is gone, its basic patterns are dissolved in nature and inclined to be reborn."[8]

Rebirth in this sense is different from a theory of reincarnation. With reincarnation, "I" get somehow incarnated in a different form or in a future life, whereas in Patañjali's reference to the body at death, he says that something continues but he does not hint at what. In other words, as the elements separate, they return to their form as basic patterns of nature.

If buried, the skin decomposes, is eaten by worms, the worms in turn die into the earth element, and out of this a flower blooms and is pollinated by bees. Or if the body is burned, the smoke from the body mixes with the earth element, as do the ashes, and the cycle of those particles continues. But what does not continue is the story of "me." So if that story, which is what is most tenuously held on to (abhiniveśa) dissolves at death, why not begin its dissolution now?

As a puzzle we can imagine it as follows: If death is inevitable, then the only thing we can change, once born, is birth. How can we change birth once we are born? By simply ceasing to construct a self through which we filter our experiences. In this way we die into life. What dies? Our "self" constructions.

When you move the body with the breath, you are meditating in action on the way the elements operate in the body. We stretch the breath through the elements in the same way that we press the breath through the kośas. Like the five elements, the kośas are perspectival glasses through which we can gain insight into the impermanent and contingent nature of the body.

When this same insight is pushed even further, especially in sitting meditation or prāṇāyāma, we see that the body in itself does not actually exist but is a coming together and coming apart of these elemental qualities. It is no longer a body but the arising and passing away of the causes and conditions of the elements. This constant transformation of the elements is described as pariṇāma. *Pariṇāma* refers to the ever-constant change and transformation of the substratum of material existence.

Human beings develop an inordinate number of strategies to fend off awareness of our mortality. It's not just the body that is immortal but also every moment of experience. Every breath, thought, action, and deed is impermanent. Ernest Becker, in his Pulitzer Prize–winning book of 1974, *The Denial of Death,* describes how our most basic activity is the creation of stories about ourselves that avoid the inevitability of facing death. "The practice of dying little by little, every day," Pattabhi Jois once said, "brings yoga."[9] Letting go in the face of death turns dying into an act of giving. Dying little by little through giving oneself completely to each and every experience describes in yogic terms how a person finds release from the anxiety and symptoms of repression that go hand in hand with a denial of change. Letting go in each moment urges us to face directly our mortality and allows an awareness of death to purify our motives.

This psychological denial of death, Becker claims, is one of the most basic drives in individual behavior, and is reflected throughout human culture. Indeed, one of the main functions of culture, according to Becker, is to help us successfully avoid awareness of our mortality. That suppression of awareness plays a crucial role in keeping people functioning—if we were constantly aware of our fragility, of the nothingness we are a split second away from at all times, we'd go insane. And how does culture perform this crucial function? By making us feel certain that we, or realities we are part of, are permanent, invulnerable, eternal. And in Becker's view, some of the personal and social consequences of this are disastrous.

As we have explored in this book, the personal and relational effects of clinging to permanence create violence, addiction, fear, and suffering. At the personal level, by ignoring our mortality and vulnerability we build up an unreal sense of self, and we act out of a false sense of who and what we are. So yoga takes us to the crucial point: the matter of letting death penetrate the self. The acceptance of death, much like being fully engaged in life, is the acceptance of the perishing of everything that will perish. In this acceptance a person imaginatively and physically experiences the process of the death of the body and the possibility of resting in the unknowability of what comes next. The next moment, even in daily life, is invisible. This body, this ability to be aware, and this precious and complex human intelligence is quite obviously not self-created but given to itself: it has emerged from the same mysterious ground as everything else. When there is attachment, we are visiting, floating, distinguishing ourselves from the ongoing interaction of life's moments. Actualized by the truth of death, we no longer need to move our lives forward shading experience according to our own ideas. When there is amazement, when there is wonder, then we are present with life and one another. And Patañjali in the *Yoga-Sutra* says that this world, this life, is here only as a phenomenal experience for us to see through it.[10]

Contemplation of death, if thought of only in the context of "me," is depressing and easily slips into nihilism. But a contemplation of death that includes the death of "me," with a heart that's open, invites us to connect with the world, and spontaneously dissolves attachment. And when attachment to our ideas about self are untangled, then automatically there is love, there is compassion. Whenever there is attachment, there is no relationship; whenever there is expectation, there is no love. Love occurs when expectation dissolves. Love is the ultimate healer in crisis, because it is letting go of our viewpoint that resolves crisis, and out of that, spontaneously, love occurs, flourishing occurs, and mokṣa occurs. Enlightenment is not someplace far away, it is right here, right now. This practice of yoga is continuously putting us in the present moment, in community. Flourishing is the opposite of nihilism, duḥkha, and the fear of death.

We contemplate death and in doing so discover our own existence to be participation in a reality that has two distinct dimensions of meaning: a dimension of things that perish, and an awareness that seems outside of that which changes. Yoga teaches us that the dance of all we perceive happens in front of awareness, not inside or behind it. Furthermore, awareness is not an "it" or anything that the mind can capture with concepts and words, and even when we rest in the idea that it is not possible to reify pure awareness, the mind comes in and does so anyway, even with terms like *puruṣa, Brahma, śūnyāta.* The "practice of dying" is a matter of learning to live the tension "in between" these two dimensions of existence. Again, human existence is not just the life of perishing existence; it is not the existence of a stone or a tree. Neither is it a life of a self-sufficient and permanent being. Human existence is a life "in between" these, participating in both because they are complementary opposites inseparable from each other.

By saying that puruṣa (pure awareness) is unchanging, Patañjali describes the human experience as not exactly bound by death, but rather informed by it. In us, the knowledge of death structures a consciousness that reaches beyond the limits of the perishable, because we come to see that even though everything perceptible is changing, that change continues in modified forms beyond any of our ideas about time. Conscious existence is not just mortality plus an extraneous dollop of intelligent awareness; it is a true union of opposites. A human life unfolds within the tenuous domains of perishing and nonperishing reality simultaneously; it is life structured by death.

In order to be authentically human, we need to accept the mystery and responsibility of participation in both of these dimensions of reality that constitute life structured by death. At the end of the day, there are not two categories of experience, only a mind that sets up two categories for explanatory purposes. The heart of yoga is the realization of the inherent flow of life within the reality of a conditional existence. This moves us to become better humans. This also returns us again to the first limb (yama) of practice: the responsibility we all share to contribute to the peace and flexibility rather than the violence and rigidity of this world. If we are to live together in this overpopulated, impermanent, and conflicted world, a meditation on death is a helpful antidote to self-centeredness. Yoga teaches us that, like jewels in Indra's Net, when we lose our sense of separateness from one another and from the world-at-large, when the conceit "I am" is seen to be nothing other than a fictional creation, we become the net.

# Acknowledgments

WITH GRATITUDE I thank the growing community of practitioners who with great enthusiasm, heart, and critical intelligence support my teaching and practice. Centre of Gravity Sangha in Toronto, a loose-knit group of yoga and Buddhist practitioners, has been central to the creation of this book. Also to my psychotherapy clients, who have taught me the value of relationship as the central factor in healing. To Gordon Thomas, who walked me through every stage of this process, which began with an unruly pile of lecture transcripts and over the course of a focused week in Cape Cod became something of a book.

Richard Freeman taught me through formal teaching as well as through his generous presence what an embodied yoga practice can become. Although I have had the opportunity to study with many teachers, a few instances marked the origination of this book: conversations with Chip Hartranft about his stellar translation of Patañjali's *Yoga-Sutra,* as well as the guiding scholarship of Christopher Chapple, David Loy, Ian Whicher, and Stephen Batchelor. Thank you also to Simone Moir and Angela Szeto for typing and formatting help. Emily Bower and the team at Shambhala have made this a better book than it would have been otherwise.

I began practicing yoga during an extraordinarily difficult phase of my life, and I thank the many teachers and guides, in both presence and written word, for showing me the possibility and example of a life well lived. The path of yoga comes alive for me in the context of family life; and the support of my partner, Michelle, and our son, Arlyn, have inspired, nurtured, and shaped everything articulated in this book.

# Notes

## Chapter 2. Embracing Suffering

1. Venkatesananda, *The Concise Yoga Vāsiṣṭa,* trans. Christopher Chapple (Albany: State University of New York Press, 1984), 9.
2. Venkatesananda, *Concise Yoga Vāsiṣṭa,* 361.
3. Pattabhi Jois, www.ayri.org/method.htm.
4. Blaise Pascal, *Pensées,* trans. A. J. Krailsheimer (London: Penguin, 1966).
5. Quoted in Donald Kalsched, *The Inner World of Trauma: Archetypal Defences of the Human Spirit* (London: Routledge, 1996), 44.
6. Venkatesananda, *Concise Yoga Vāsiṣṭa,* 361.
7. Carl Jung, *Mysterium Coniunctionus, Collected Works 14* (Princeton, N.J.: Princeton University Press, 1955), par. 151.
8. Sigmund Freud, "Remembering, Repeating, and Working-through" [1914], in *Standard Edition of the Complete Psychological Works of Sigmund Freud,* ed. and trans. James Strachey (London: Hogarth Press, 1966).

## Chapter 3. *Mārga*

1. "The Dynamics of Transference," *The Standard Edition of the Complete Psychological Works of Sigmund Freud,* trans. James Strachey, vol. 12 (1911–1913) (London: Hogarth Press, 1966), 113.

## Chapter 4. Embodying the Path

1. Czeslaw Milosz quoted in Jane Hirshfield, "Poetry, Zazen and the Net of Connection," in *Beneath A Single Moon,* ed. Kent Johnson and Craig Paulenich (Boston: Shambhala Publications, 1991), 152.
2. The *Yoga-Sutra* attributed to Patañjali, chap. 1, line 12, Chip Hartranft, trans. (Boston: Shambhala Publications, 2003).
3. Borges, Jorge Luis, *Selected Poems, 1923–1967* (London: Penguin, 1985), 441.
4. *The Principal Upanishads,* ed. and trans. S. Radhakrishnan (London: George Allen & Unwin, 1953), *Chāndogya Upaniṣad* 6.8.1–2.

5. John Cage.
6. *Mahabarata,* vol. 1, translated by Ishvar Chandra Sharma and O. M. Bimali (Delhi: Parimal Publishing, 2006).
7. Stephen Mitchell, *Bhagavad Gita: A New Translation* (New York: Three Rivers Press, 2000), 12.
8. Irvin Yalom, quoted in Ken Wilber, *Spectrum of Consciousness* (Wheaton, Ill.: Theosophical Publishing House, 1997), 123.

## Chapter 5. The Eight Limbs

1. Virginia Woolf, *The Diary of Virginia Woolf,* ed. Anne Olivier and consultant ed. Andrew McNeillie (New York: Harcourt, 1985), 224.
2. Richard Freeman, "Glossary of Terms" (teacher training handout, Yoga Workshop, Boulder, 2002).

## Chapter 6. Practicing the *Yamas*

1. Patañjali, *The Yoga-Sutra of Patañjali,* trans. Chip Hartranft (Boston: Shambhala Publications, 2003), 103.
2. Hilary Putnam quoted in Adam Philips, *Terrors and Experts* (Cambridge, Mass.: Harvard University Press, 1995), 92.
3. Mohandas Gandhi, *Sarvodaya (The Welfare of All),* ed. Bharatan Kumarappa (Ahmedabad, India: Navajivan, 1954), 12.
4. *Meditations,* Shambhala Classics edition (Boston: Shambhala Publications, 2002).
5. Based on the Mindfulness Training of the Order of Interbeing, originally written by Thich Nhat Hanh: "Any form of sexual relation motivated by craving cannot dissipate the feelings of loneliness or longing. . . ." Thich Nhat Hanh, *Interbeing: Fourteen Guidelines for Engaged Buddhism* (Berkeley, Calif.: Parallax Press, 1999), 40.
6. Ibid.
7. Patañjali, *The Yoga-Sutra of Patañjali: A New Translation and Commentary,* trans. Georg Feuerstein (Rochester, N.Y.: Inner Traditions International, 1989).

## Chapter 7. The *Yamas* Beyond Dualism

1. Wendy Doniger O'Flaherty, trans., *The Rig-Veda: An Anthology* (London: Penguin, 1981), 9.113.7.

## Chapter 8. The Five *Kleṣas*

1. Kabir, *The Kabir Book,* ed. and trans. Robert Bly (New York: Beacon Press, 1971), 50.

## CHAPTER 9. FREEDOM THROUGH THE *KLEŚAS*

1. Heinz Kohut, *The Resoration of the Self* (New York: International Universities Press, 1977), 310–11.
2. "Krishna Story Boy" in *Rig-Veda,* trans. Wendy Doniger (London: Penguin Classics, 1981).
3. Luce Irigaray, *je, tous, nous: Toward a Culture of Difference* (New York: Routledge, 1993), 38-40.
4. Ibid., 39.
5. Ibid.
6. Wallace Stevens, *Opus Posthumous* (New York: Vintage Books, 1957), 189.

## CHAPTER 10. STILLNESS AND MOVEMENT

1. Erich Schiffmann, *Yoga: The Spirit and Practice of Moving into Stillness* (New York: Pocket Books, 1996), 1.
2. Sankaracarya, *Aparokshanubhuti,* trans. Richard Freeman, line 114. (personal communication). See also *Complete Works of Sankarcharya* in the original Sanskrit, in *Miscellaneous Prakaranas,* vol. 2 (Madras, India: Samata Books, 1981), 215–33.

## CHAPTER 11. THE FIVE *KOŚAS*: SHEATHS OF THE MIND-BODY

1. B.K.S. Iyengar, *Light on Prāṇayama* (New York: Crossroad Publishing, 1999), 8-9.

## CHAPTER 12. WORKING WITH THE *KOŚAS*

1. I am indebted to Stephen Batchelor's idea of compartmentalizing a "me inside a body inside a world," and for helping me to articulate these ideas. It was a retreat with him, when he presented the notions of torment and anguish through compartmentalizing aspects of the self, that opened up for me a new way of understanding duḥkha.

## CHAPTER 13. *SAṀSKĀRAS*: WEBS OF MIND AND BODY

1. Swatmarama, *Hatha Yoga Pradipika* (Madras, India: Adyar Library and Research Centre, 1975), 7.

## CHAPTER 14. *PRĀṆA:* ENERGETIC FLOW

1. Robert Wright, *The Moral Animal* (New York: Pantheon, 1994), 77.

## Chapter 15. Body in Mind

1. *Yoga-Sutra,* attributed to Patañjali, 1.9, trans. Chip Hartranft (Boston: Shambhala Publications, 2003).

## Chapter 16. Letting Go: *Āsana* and Meditation Intertwined

1. *Chandogya Upaniṣad* in *The Upanishads,* trans. Valerie Roebuck (London: Penguin Classics, 2004).
2. *Yoga Sutra of Patanjali* 2.46–54, my own translation.
3. Wendy Doniger O'Flaherty, *Dreams, Illusions and Other Realities* (Chicago: University of Chicago Press, 1984), 273.
4. Christopher Chapple, Introduction to *The Concise Yoga Vāsiṣṭha,* trans. Swami Venkatesananda (Albany, N.Y.: SUNY, 1984), ix.

## Chapter 17. *Prāṇa* and *Citta*

1. B.K.S. Iyengar, *The Tree of Yoga: Yoga Vrksa* (Boston: Shambhala Publications, 1989), 4–5.
2. Venkatesananda, *The Concise Yoga Vāsiṣṭa,* trans. Christopher Chapple (Albany: State University of New York Press, 1984), 238.
3. Ibid.
4. T.K.V. Desikachar, *The Heart of Yoga* (Rochester, Vt.: Inner Traditions International, 1998), 140.
5. Ibid.
6. Swami Rama, *Lectures on Yoga* (Honesdale, Pa.: Himalayan International Institute, 1979), 93.
7. B.K.S. Iyengar, *Light on Yoga* (London: Thorsons/HarperCollins, 2001), 37.

## Chapter 18. The Empty Vessel

1. Li Po, "Zazen on Ching-t'ing Mountain," in *Crossing the Yellow River: Three Hundred Poems from the Chinese*, trans. Sam Hamill (Rochester, N.Y.: BOA Editions, 2000), 44.
2. Robert Thurman, *Yoga and Buddhism,* audio recording of lecture at Jivamukti Yoga Studio, New York, 1999.
3. Yājñavalka story quoted in David Loy, *Nonduality* (New Haven: Yale University Press, 1988), 198.
4. Ibid.
5. Patañjali, *The Yoga-Sutra of Patañjali,* trans. Chip Hartranft (Boston: Shambhala Publications, 2003), 22.
6. Marcel Proust, *In Search of Lost Time,* vol. 2, *Within a Budding Grove,* trans. D. J. Everett, C. K. Scott Moncrieff, and Terence Kilmartin (New York: Modern Library/Random House, 1998).

7. Stephen Batchelor, *Buddhism and Postmodernity,* www.stephenbatchelor.org/online%20articles/buddhism%20postmodernity.htm.
8. Adyanshanti, *Radical Emptiness,* www.adyashanti.org/index.php?file=writings_inner&writingid=26.

## Chapter 19. *Śūnyatā:* Boundless and Empty

1. R. C. Zaehner, *Mysticism: Sacred and Profane* (Oxford, Eng.: Clarendon Press, 1957), 127.
2. "Happy are those who know," by Rainer Maria Rilke, trans. Jane Hirshfield, in *Beneath A Single Moon: Buddhism in Contemporary American Poetry,* ed. Kent Johnson (Boston: Shambhala Publications, 1991).
3. Wendy Doniger O'Flaherty, trans., *The Rig-Veda: An Anthology* (London: Penguin, 1981), 10.129.6.
4. Ibid.
5. Ibid.
6. Patañjali, *The Yoga-Sutra of Patañjali,* trans. Chip Hartranft (Boston: Shambhala Publications, 2003), 112.
7. Sri Nisargadatta Maharaj, *The Nectar of Immortality: Sri Nisargadatta Maharaj's Discourses on the Eternal,* ed. Robert Powell (San Diego: Blue Dove Press, 1987), 44.
8. Don Cupitt, "Learning to Live with One Foot in the Grave," *Face to Faith,* December 1993, www.sofn.org.uk/The_Collection/The_Guardian/ofigrave.html.
9. Venkatesananda, *The Concise Yoga Vāsiṣṭa,* trans. Christopher Chapple (Albany: State University of New York Press, 1984), 361.

## Chapter 20. Yoga, Death, and Dying: What Is Most Astounding?

1. This is my own translation of the *Śrimadbhāgavatamahāpuranā,* book 16, chap. 6, ed. Kṛṣṇaśaṅkaraḥ at. 12 vols. (Vārāṇasi, India: Saṁsāra Press, Vim. Sam, 2002).
2. Cindy Carroll, personal communication, 2006.
3. *The Heart of Awareness: A Translation of the Ashtavakra Gita,* trans. Thomas Byrom (Boston: Shambhala Publications, 1990), 28.
4. Raymond Carver, "Late Fragment," in *A Path to the Waterfall* (New York: The Atlantic Monthly Press, 1989), 122.
5. Joan Halifax, *Being with Dying: Cultivating Compassion and Fearlessness in the Presence of Death* (Boston: Shambhala Publications, 2008); personal communication, 2006.
6. E. H. Jarrow, *Tales for the Dying: The Death Narrative of the Bhagavata Purana* (Albany: State University of New York Press, 2003), 162.

7. Don Cupitt, "Learning to Live with One Foot in the Grave," *Face to Faith,* December 1993, www.sofn.org.uk/The_Collection/The_Guardian/ofigrave.html.
8. Patañjali, *The Yoga-Sutra of Patañjali,* my own translation.
9. Personal communication, 2000.
10. The Yoga Sutra of Patañjali, 4.15–26, my own translation.

# Glossary of Sanskrit Terms

**abhiniveśa** Self-preservation; instinctive clinging to life and the fear that one may be cut off from all by death; will to live; strong desire; fear of letting go of the stories of "I, me, and mine."

**abhyāsa** Practice; action; method; continuous endeavor; repetition; exercise; exertion. From the verb root "as," meaning *to throw,* plus "abhi," meaning *toward.*

**advaita** Nondualism; nonduality. Literally "not two," from "a," meaning *not,* plus "dvaita," meaning *dual* or *two.*

**Agni** Fire. A Vedic god

**ahaṇkāra** The concept of individuality, from the verb root "kṛ," meaning *action,* plus "aham," meaning *I*); ego or egoism; literally "the I-maker," the state that ascertains "I know"; "I-maker," source of egoism; the sense that identification is occurring.

**ahiṁsā** Not harming; non-injury; nonviolence. From the verb root "hiṁs," meaning *to injure,* plus the prefix "a," meaning *not.* The word has not merely the negative and restrictive meaning of "nonkilling" or "nonviolence," but the positive and comprehensive meaning of "love embracing all creation."

**ānanda** Bliss; joy; delight; a type of samādhi. From the verb root "nand," meaning *to rejoice.*

**ānandamaya kośa** The sheath (kośa) of joy or bliss (ānanda) enveloping the ātman; the felt sense of everything being OK.

**anātman** With substance; non-self. From "an," meaning *not,* plus "ātman," meaning *self.*

**annamaya kośa** The sheath of food.

**apana** "Carrying-downwards breath"; inspired breath; outbreath; exhalation;

digestive energy. From the root "an," meaning *to breath,* plus "apa," meaning *away*. The downward, contracting, rooting movement characteristic of exhaling. It is based at the center of the perineum, the Mūladhāra Chakra. Apān is said to tether prāṇa. The inner experience of hatha yoga begin by consciously uniting prāṇa with apāna, to feel their actions within each other.

**aparigraha** Nonpossession, nongrasping; nondesiring; not greedy; not being acquisitive; freedom from hoarding or collecting.

**āsana** Posture; seat; to "sit with."

**asmitā** The sense of "I," egoism; the state of concentration; an impurity.

**asteya** Not stealing.

**aṣṭāṅga** Literally, "Eight Limbs." Refers to a yoga practice that leads to deep, spontaneous meditation and complete liberation. The variety of limbs guarantees that the awareness operates in all spheres of one's life, so that no distortion, perversion, or fantasy will attempt to usurp the solid ground of real yogic insight. In many of the Yoga Upaniṣads the eight limbs are further expanded into fifteen. The advantage of considering the path of yoga to have many aspects is that one is encouraged not to neglect the moral, the ethical, the interpersonal, the physiological, the esoteric, and the meditative aspects of practice. The term *aṣṭāṅga* implies both a simultaneous realization of all these interrelated aspects of practice and a logical step by step progression in which one limb prepares one to truly practice the next one.

**atha** The present moment, a term used to express a beginning; doubt; interrogation; condition; "after, then, now."

**ātman** The inner self. "Ātma" means "breath," from the verb root "at," meaning *to breathe,* or "āp," meaning *to pervade* or *reach up to.*

**avidyā** Not seeing things as they are; lack of wisdom, ignorance of one's true nature; from the root verb "vid," meaning *to know*, plus the prefix "a," meaning *not*.

**bandha** Bond; valve; control; determination. From the verb root "bandh," meaning *to bind.*

**bhakti** Loving devotion. From the verb root "bhajj," meaning *to love, worship, revere.*

**bhūta** Element; gross elemental principle. From the verb root "bhū," meaning *to become* or *to exist.*

**bhujaṅga** Cobra.

**Brahmā** The creator of the universe; one of the Indian trinity comprising Brahmā, Viṣṇu, and Rudra.

**brahmacharya** Wise use of sexual energy; a code of conduct; dwelling in Brahman; a student; "the path that leads to Brahman" or "moving in Brahman"; a life of celibacy, religious study and self-restraint; impeccable conduct.

**buddhi** Intellect; the discriminative faculty; perception. From the verb root "budh," meaning *to enlighten, to know.*

**buddhindriyas** Sense capacities, i.e., hearing, feeling, seeing, tasting and smelling.

**chakra** Wheel or circle; center; disc; plexus; centers in the body; energy center. From the verb root "car," meaning *to move.*

**citta** Consciousness; where name and form meet. From the verb root "cit," meaning *to perceive, to observe, to think, to be aware,* or *to know.*

**dhāraṇā** Meditation; support; single-mindedness; "holding bearing"; to keep in remembrance.

**dhyāna** Concentration.

**duḥkha** Unsatisfaction; lack; distress; suffering; sorrow; that which is unsatisfactory (because it is impermanent). From "dur," meaning *bad,* plus "kha," meaning *state.*

**dveṣa** Antipathy; hatred; aversion. From the verb root "dviś," meaning *to hate.*

**garuḍa** Eagle; Viṣṇu's vehicle; "devourer."

**granthi** Knot. From the root "granth," meaning *to string together.*

**guna** Quality; attribute; characteristic; excellence; rope; constituent; subsidiary; mode; fundamental quality of nature.

**guru** Teacher; preceptor; great; mentor; heavy; weighty; venerable. From the verb root "gṛ," meaning *to invoke* or *to praise.*

**hālāhala** Poisonous herb; metaphor for samsara.

**iḍā nadi** The psychic nerve or tube on the right side of the spine; a nādī or channel of energy starting from the left nostril, then moving under the crown of the head and thence descending to the root of the spine. In its course it conveys lunar energy and is therefore called Chandra nadi (channel of lunar energy).

**Indra** Ruler; chief (of the gods in the Vedic pantheon); mighty; powerful.

**īśvara-pranidhānā** Devotion to a god; divine ideal of pure awareness (īśvara); surrender; dedication (praṇidhānāt).

**jīva** Invidual soul; life; embodied self; living entity. From the verb root "jīv," meaning *to live.*

**jñāna** Knowledge; wisdom; insight; comprehension. From the verb roon "jñā," meaning *to know.*

**kaivalya** The distinct difference between puruṣa, meaning pure awareness, and prakṛti, meaning all changing phenomena; emancipation; isolation of pure awareness.

**kāma** Desire; pleasure; lust; love. From the verb root "kām," meaning *to desire.*

**kapota** Dove or pigeon.

**karma** Volitional action and result; creativity; rite; deed; cause and effect; accumulation of past actions; physical, verbal, or mental action. From the verb root "kṛ," meaning *to act, to do,* or *to make.*

**karmedriyas** Action capacities, i.e., speaking, holding, walking, excreting, and procreating.

**karuṇā** Compassion.

**kleṣa** Cause of suffering; corruption; hindrance; affliction; poison; passion; defiling element. From the verb root "kliś," meaning *to torment* or *distress.*

**kośa** Sheath; cover; subtle body; treasury; lexicon. From the root "kuś," meaning *to enfold.*

**krodha** Anger; wrathful; furious. From the verb root "krudh," meaning *to be angry.*

**kuṇḍalinī** Serpent; life force; a type of yoga; coiled; winding; spiraled; "coiled one." From the verb root "kuṇḍ," meaning *to burn.* The burning up of knots and holding patterns in mind and body, the most significant of which is the clinging to self-image.

**lobha** Greed; covetousness.

**mada** Pride; conceit; intoxication; exhilaration; dementia.

**mahābhūta** The five gross material elements, i.e., space, wind, fire, water, air, and earth.

**maṇḍala** Circle; magic circle; the special domain of any particular divinity; energy cycle; a section of the Ṛg Veda.

**manomaya kośa** One of the sheaths (kośa) covering the atman; the sheath of the mind, the manomaya kośa affects the functions of awareness, feeling, and motivation not derived from subjective experience.

**mārga** Way; path; street. From the verb root "mārg," meaning *to seek, to strive.*

**mātsarya** Envy; jealousy.

**māyā** The principle of appearance; illusion; marvelous power of creation; magical power; mystery; "that which measures." From the verb root "mā," meaning *to measure, to limit, give form.*

**moha** Infatuation; delusion. From the verb root "muh," meaning *to delude.*

**mokṣa** Liberation; spiritual freedom; release; final emancipation of the ātman from recurring births. From the verb root "mokṣ," meaning *to liberate.*

**mṛtyu** Death; to grind down.

**mūla bandha** Mūla root. Primary, original, text; the natural and spontaneous contraction of the perineal muscles and the drawing of the attention to its center point just in front of the anus and behind the genitals. It is essentially a meditative awakening at what it feels to be like at the root of the body (the mūla), done in conjunction with the breath.

**nadi** River; nerve; vessel; ducts for vital air ("prāṇa"); conduit; energy channel; vein; artery.

**nama** Name.

**neti, neti** Not this not this (not such, not such). From "na," meaning *not,* plus "iti," meaning *thus.*

**nirodha** Stilling; negation; cessation; restriction. From the root verb "rudh," meaning *to obstruct, arrest, avert,* plus "ni," meaning *down* or *into.*

**nirvāna** Extinction; perfection; the Great Peace; literally "blowing out," from the verb root "vā," meaning *to blow* plus "nir," meaning *out.*

**niyamas** Internal discipline.

**padmāsana** Lotus posture.

**paramātman** The supreme self; Brahman; God; the Absolute; the selfless self of awareness. From "parama," meaning *highest,* plus "ātman," meaning *self.*

**pariṇāma** Change; modification; transformation; evolution; development; ripening; changing; the ever-constant change and transformation of the substratum of material existence.

**piṅgalā** A nadi or channel of energy, starting from the right nostril, then moving to the crown of the head and thence downwards to the base of the spine. As the solar energy flows through it, it is also call sūrya nadi (Sun channel). Piṅgalā means *tawny* or *reddish.*

**prāṇamaya kośa** The sheath of vital air; the physiological (prāṇamaya) sheath (kośa), which along with the psychological (manomaya) and intellectual (vijñānamaya) sheaths, make up the subtle body (sūkṣma srira enveloping the ātman. The prāṇamaya kośa includes the respiratory, circulatory, digestive, endocrine, excretory and genital systems.

**prajāpati** Lord of creatures; creator; lord of becoming. From "prajā," meaning *creation,* plus "pati," meaning *lord.*

**prajñā** Wisdom; intuitive wisdom; gnosis.

**prakṛti** Primal nature; primordial nature; phenomenal world; creatrix. From the verb root "kṛ," meaning *to make* or *to do,* plus "pra," meaning *forth.*

**prāṇa** Vital air; life breath; vitality; the upward, expanding, blossoming movement characteristic of inhaling. From the verb root "an," meaning *to breathe,* plus "pra," meaning *forth.* It is said to be centered in the Anāhata Chakra (heart center); Apān is said to tether prāṇa. Yoga begins by consciously uniting prāṇa with apāna, to feel their actions within each other.

**prana vāyuu** A breath cycle with attention to the internal pattern of inhaling.

**prāṇāyāma** Control of breath; breath regulation; restraint of the breath.

**pratyāhāra** The natural uncoupling of sense organs and sense objects during concentration; withdrawal of the senses from their objects; beyond the mind.

**pṛthvī** The earth.

**purāṇa** Ancient; old; folk tales or Indian teachings. From the verb root "pur," meaning *to go before* or *to precede.*

**puruṣa** Pure awareness; cosmic person.

**raga** Wanting; desire; passion; attachment.

**rāja** Royal; king. From the verb root "rāj," meaning *to reign,* or *illuminate.*

**rodha** To hold or keep a check on something; the goddess of storms.

**śāstra** Scripture; teaching; doctrine; treatise. From the verb root "śās," meaning *to rule* or *to teach.*

**Śākti** Power; capacity; energy; potency; "citi" or "kuṇḍalinī"; force, the divine cosmic energy which projects, maintains and dissolves the universive; the spouse of Śiva (from "śak"= to be able); female energy.

**śauca** Purity; cleanliness.

**sahasrāra** The thousand-petaled; the seventh subtle center.

**saṁsāra** Empirical existence; the wheel of birth and death; transmigration; the flux of the world; the flow of the world; the objective universe; this world; worldly illusion. From the verb root "sṛ," meaning *to flow* plus "sam," meaning *together.*

**saṁskāra** Psycho-physical grooves; latent impression; predisposition; consecration; imprint; innate tendency; innate potence; mold; inborn nature; residual impression; purificatory rite; rite of passage. From"sam," plus "kṛ," meaning *to fashion* or *to do together*.

**saṁyoga** Conjunction; contact; coupling; union; association; mingling.

**samādhi** One-pointedness; oneness; concentration; integration; absorption; union; a calm, desireless fixity; unifying concentration; "equal mind." From the verb root "dhā," meaning *to hold*, plus the prefixes "ā" and "sam," meaning *together completely*.

**samstitihi** Equal standing.

**santoṣa** Contentment; peace.

**satya** Honesty; truthfulness; truth. From the verb root "as," meaning *to be*.

**śavāsanā** Corpse pose.

**Śiva** Auspicious; the Ultimate Reality; Lord; male energy.

**skandha** Group; aggregate.

**smṛti** Memory; recollection; depth memory; "that which is remembered"; immediate attention; mindfulness with the following attributes in mature practice: present-centered, nonconceptual, nonjudgmental, intentional, engaged through nonattachment, nonverbal, exploratory, liberating, steady, and at ease. From the verb root "smṛ," meaning *to remember*.

**śūnya** Boundlessness; empty; zero. From the verb root "śū" or "śva" or śvi," meaning *to swell.*

**śūnyatā** Insubstantiality; emptiness.

**suṣumnā nadi** The subtle central nerve; the principal nerve; the main channel of energy situated in the spinal column.

**sūtra** Aphorism; thread; condensed mnemonic verse. From the verb root "siv," meaning *to sew*.

**svādhyāya** Self-study; education of the self; reflection. From "sva," meaning *self*, plus the verb root "adhi-i," meaning *to go over*.

**svarūpa** Natural form; actual or essential nature; essence; own form, identity. From "sva," meaning *own* or *self*, plus "rūpa," meaning *form, shape,* or *figure*.

**tanmātra** The subtle essence of the fire elements; the pure elements; the subtle elements, namely, the essence of sound (śabda), touch (sparśa), form (rūpa), flavor (rasa) and odor (gandha). They are subtle objects of the sense powers (indriyas), namely, the powers of hearing (śrota), feeling (tvak), seeing (chaksu), tasting (rasanā) and smelling (ghrāna).

**tantra** Rule; ritual; scripture; religious treatise; loom; warp. From the root "tan," meaning *to do in detail,* plus "trā," meaning *to protect.*

**tapas** Heat; intensity of discipline; concentrated discipline; austerity; penance; energy; to heat up. From the verb root "tap," meaning *to burn.*

**vāsanā** Latent tendency; impression; conditioning; self-limitation; predisposition; desires. Also called saṁskāra.

**vāyuu** Air; life breath; the wind; the vital airs.

**vairāgya** Dispassion; detachment; renunciation; nonattachment; absence of worldly desires.

**vajra** Thunderbolt; diamond.

**vidyā** Knowledge; meditation; wisdom; insight.

**vijñanamaya kośa** The sheath of intelligence, affecting the process of reasoning and judgment derived from subjective experience.

**vinyasa** A sequence, connoting a step-by-step progression from one stage to another. This is how all things evolve in natural systems. Like a sprout bursting up and sinking roots in complete symbiosis with time, temperature, soil air and light; so yoga postures and meditative insights are part of a singular system which works from within the space of pure intelligence.

**vipāka** Effect of an action; a type of transformation; ripening, resultant; fruition.

**virāsana** Hero's pose.

**Viṣṇu** The supreme Lord; the all-pervading; the spirit of time.

**viveka** Discrimination.

**vṛtti** Mental mode; a modification of the mind whose function is to manifest objects; being; condition; fluctuation; activity; patternings, turnings, movements. From the verb root "vṛt," meaning *to turn, revolve, roll, move.*

**yama** Abstention; self-control; restraint; external discipline. From "yam," meaning *to restrain.*

**yuj** To unite; join; connect.

# Permissions

"Happy are those who know," by Rainer Maria Rilke, translated by Jane Hirshfield © 1988 Jane Hirshfield, used by permission of Jane Hirshfield. First appeared in *Beneath a Single Moon: Buddhism in Contemporary American Poetry,* edited by Kent Johnson. Boston: Shambhala Publications, 1991.

"Friend" by Kabir, translated by Robert Bly. From *The Kabir Book,* edited by Robert Bly. Boston: Beacon Press, 1977. Reprinted with permission, Beacon Press, Boston.

Li Po, "Zazen on Ching-t'ing Mountain," from *Crossing the Yellow River: Three Hundred Poems from the Chinese,* translated by Sam Hamill. Copyright © 2000 Sam Hamill. Reprinted with the permission of BOA Editions, Ltd.

# Index